Peace *in the* Storm

Peace in the Storm

A Journey with Cancer
– THE SHIRLEY DANDO STORY –

By the Dando Family *with Lynette Davies*

Peace in the Storm
Published by Graeme Dando
New Zealand

© 2019 Graeme Dando

ISBN 978-0-473-50219-5 (Softcover)
ISBN 978-0-473-50220-1 (ePUB)
ISBN 978-0-473-50221-8 (Kindle)

Writing:
Lynette Davies in consultation with
Graeme Dando and Michelle McCarter

Production & Typesetting:
Andrew Killick
Castle Publishing Services
www.castlepublishing.co.nz

Cover design:
Paul Smith

Bible copyright and other permissions
are recorded in the end pages of this book.

ALL RIGHTS RESERVED

No part of this publication may be reproduced,
stored in a retrieval system, or transmitted
in any form or by any means, electronic, mechanical,
photocopying, recording or otherwise,
without prior written permission from the publisher.

Contents

	Preface	7
	Introduction	9
1	An Uncharted Path	13
2	Stark Reality	31
3	Wonderful Partnership	51
4	Quality Time	71
5	Shattered Plans	83
6	Reality of Faith	93
7	A New Diagnosis	113
8	Wonderful Respite	133
9	Appreciating Each Other	147
10	Treatment Concluded	169
11	Time Out	187
12	Rays of Light	207
13	Why Me, Lord?	225
14	Tried as by Fire	241
	Epilogue	253
	Dear Reader	257
	Glossary of Terms	259

Preface

When asked to consider this project, my initial reaction after reading Shirley's journal was to wonder whether people would want to read about so much suffering without the consolation of a traditional happy ending. But I slept on it and woke the next morning with words forming in my head, demanding to be written.

I realised that the spaces in Shirley's journal were sometimes more revealing than the written entries. Those were the times when she was either struggling to come to terms with what was happening to her; or she was experiencing a period of respite and was afraid to validate it only to have her hopes dashed. So she drew instead on her daily readings and found sustenance in the words of others. The verses she chose were a reflection of where she was at emotionally – they were, in effect, her mood barometer.

It was Shirley's unspoken voice that convinced me her story needed to be told. I felt that it would be a tragedy if this wonderful passionate woman, with such generosity of spirit, was to be ultimately defined by her illness. Snippets of her vibrant personality and quirky sense of humour sprinkled throughout her emails and journal hinted at the strength of character which enabled her to put a positive spin on everything that happened to her. She contributed much to the lives of those she touched, and will be sorely missed.

Shirley was a trained nurse and although she gave up her career to bring up her family, she retained her interest in the medical profession. Clearly this background enabled her to maintain a degree of objectivity. Often, she coped by focusing on the medical aspects of her disease and treated herself with the same detachment required when nursing a patient. She had mastered the art of being compassionate without being overwhelmed by emotion.

However, she was not alone in this journey and whenever she felt unable to carry on, she was sustained by her unwavering faith in God and the knowledge that He would not abandon her. Her relationship with God was not conditional on being completely healed on this plane. Instead she compartmentalised each stage of her journey and accepted with humble gratitude the many lesser healings and blessings she received along the way.

It has been a privilege and honour to become involved with this lovely family and share their intimate stories about Shirley. I consider her legacy to be the delightful children she left behind – Michelle and Richard are both shaped by her strong influence and have inherited her strength of character and personal integrity.

Lynette Davies

Introduction

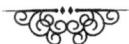

A few days after a routine mammogram, my wife Shirley received a phone call from BreastScreen Aotearoa to say that a 'shadow' had been detected and further investigation was required. Although concerned, she wasn't overly anxious as she had been reassured that dense tissue and tenderness was normal at her age. Next day, however, during an ultrasound, a 'dark spot' was located deep in her left breast and biopsies were immediately undertaken.

That was Thursday 3 June 2010. A day that will forever mark the end of life as we knew it. The day that cancer entered our lives and thrust us mercilessly into uncharted territory, on a pathway strewn with seemingly overwhelming hardship and pain, which would test our faith and throw all that we believed into contention.

We didn't doubt for one instant that anything we could experience would ever shift our intrinsic belief in our Lord and our commitment to follow His wishes in every aspect of our lives. But we were unprepared for the fact that we would become a living experiment by which others measured their own faith. We were supported or maligned, in equal measure, by friends and church members who watched from the sidelines and either expected Shirley to abide by God's will and accept her fate; or demonstrate the power of unquestioning faith and prayer so they could bear witness to a miracle.

For the duration of her journey, Shirley grappled with the conflicting paradigms of belief represented by people whose opinion she valued, and her own humility of spirit, which insisted that she question her own judgement at all times. On the one hand was the belief (substantiated by particular scriptures) that 'if we ask we shall receive' and that God would therefore heed our prayers and heal her; and the other perspective that her illness was God's will and she should submit: 'Your will, Lord, not mine.' It was a conundrum which troubled her to the very end.

Although she was a strong-minded woman, Shirley was respectful of other opinions and always remained open to differing points of view. But in illness we are at our most vulnerable so the continuous barrage of conflicting ideologies kept her constantly re-examining her own long-held beliefs. As a result, Shirley was often left struggling with her interpretation of scriptures and second-guessing her close dialogue with God.

She did not, however, waver in her trust in God and acceptance that her *days were written and she was cradled in His arms*. With every false hope, every up and every down, through pain and sorrow, laughter and tears, she continued to praise God and give thanks for each morsel of relief and small victory along the way. It was a belief that sustained her and enabled her to focus always on the glass half full and refuse to be cowed by any other perspective.

Paradoxically, rather than shake her faith, this harrowing journey strengthened her relationship with God and brought her a greater comfort and understanding than she could ever have comprehended. With every fibre of her being, she believed she was not alone. She took each step with God at her side, and when she was too weak, He carried her.

Shirley kept a private journal to document her medical procedures, as well as personal thoughts and inspirational quotes. She also maintained a more public record through regular emails, sent at the request of friends who wanted to be kept up to date so that they could support her with focused prayer. Her words in this book are taken from those two sources. As a family, we wanted to share Shirley's story in an effort to bring some solace and understanding to others going through a similar experience. Our prayer is that they will be encouraged to seek the peace that a relationship with God can bring so that they can discover for themselves the richness and blessings of living in harmony with Christ. It is some small consolation to think that her suffering was not therefore in vain.

Personally, I think it is important to show that regardless of whether we get physical healing or not, we can draw close to God, know His power and purpose, and experience His presence. As humans, we desire and seek healing in a physical form, while God desires a relationship and devotion first and foremost to Him. It is also vital to record the many situations God intervened in, even if the ultimate physical healing on earth was not granted. Simultaneously, we need to explore the other side of the Christian spectrum that says you only have to pray and ask in faith to be healed; and if you aren't healed, then you must have transgressed in some way and be unworthy.

Strongly opposed beliefs usually find a balance somewhere in between – the reality is that Jesus does heal in the 'here and now', and on other occasions He chooses to complete the healing in heaven.

I want to demonstrate through Shirley's story that it is possible to die graciously, without losing one grain of faith. Shirley lived life to the full – she was effervescent, outgoing, sociable and had boundless love and compassion for anyone in need. She remained true to her essence through the most trying times and accepted small victories along the way as answers to her prayers. Shirley was not afraid of dying (although she didn't want to die yet) but accepted that God had ordained the number of her days.

Shirley herself says it best in this excerpt from her journal:

> There is no change in my stake in the ground. I believe that a physical healing will have little effect on my relationship with God. For most of my Christian life my relationship with God has *not* been dependent on what He could do for me but rather on *who He is* and *what He has already done for me at the cross*. At its very core, my relationship is founded on an unshakeable personal awareness and knowledge of the goodness and incomprehensible love of my Heavenly Father; the sure and certain knowledge that Jesus is my Saviour and Lord; and that I have the hope of living in eternity with Him. That won't change regardless of my circumstances.

So this book has become a compilation of Shirley's own words and a chronicle of my journey as a companion to an amazing woman whom I have loved since the moment we met and planned to end my days with.

Graeme Dando
Auckland, New Zealand
October 2015

CHAPTER 1

An Uncharted Path

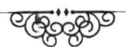

June 2010

Graeme ~ The morning prior to Shirley's first operation was filled with optimism. We woke to a strong bar of sunlight beaming through our bedroom drapes and looked out at a cloudless blue sky heralding a perfect winter's day. Although I knew that Shirley had tossed and turned throughout the night, I respected her obvious need to behave as if this was just a normal morning, so I followed her lead and adopted a cheerful demeanour. As usual we began our day with a prayer and as we both completed our contemplation, we glanced at each other and smiled. Our relaxed faces, freed from the tension that had previously held us so tightly in its grip, were a mirror of each other. We had handed it all over to God.

We had waited an interminable anxiety-filled six days for the breast biopsy results: a 1.2 centimetre malignant growth. Despite the negative outcome, we were reassured that very early diagnosis would bring with it a good outcome. For both of us, this would prove to be a challenging time, and in hindsight we were blessed in our ignorance, unaware that we had just taken the first faltering step in a macabre dance with cancer where the routines were forever changing. Meanwhile, we felt God's strong presence and an amazing peace, and believing in God's healing power, we trusted Him for the best outcome.

Knowing Shirley wanted to have her operation as soon as possible, the surgeon went ahead and booked it for the following Friday. An ultrasound was arranged prior to surgery for final marking of the lump, and we were optimistic that it may have already responded to the volume of prayer and disappeared.

Once we had absorbed the enormity of the possibilities we were now facing – that this was no casual illness which would run its course and leave no trace when it had passed – we discussed the impact on our children and how much we should share with them at this stage. Michelle and Richard were involved with university projects and Shirley was adamant we shouldn't burden them with an added stress that could impact their study. So we settled on a superficial discussion about the biopsy and possible results, but didn't emphasise our concerns. We attempted to continue living our life (on the surface at least) as normal and refused to examine the dark shadow lurking in the background.

Shirley – A sickening fear had set in. The thought of cancer overwhelmed me with panic. Most nights I slept fitfully, waking abruptly, feeling nauseated and afraid. Last night at about 1 a.m. I woke with the terrifying feeling that I was being suffocated by a large black cape stretched over my shoulders and back, restricting my breathing. My heart was racing and I was hyperventilating. Then the heaviness lifted and I felt the calming assurance of God's presence. A voice asked me: 'Do you choose life or death?' I instantly recalled careless words spoken and fleeting thoughts that my family would be better off without me; and recent prayers when I had asked God to do 'anything' necessary to bring our children into a close relationship with Him.

However, now that I was being called to account there was no hesitation: I choose life. I want to be there for Graeme, I want to be there for Michelle and Richard and share their future. I asked God's forgiveness and said emphatically, 'I want to live.' God repeated the question four times: 'Do you choose life or death?'

An exciting thing about this is that 'the spirit of death' could have no power over me because I am a child of the King of Kings. I knew His voice and was able to respond clearly and be freed from Satan's clutch. Feeling okay again, I got out of bed and went into the lounge to process the experience. I realised my previous words were in effect 'suicidal' ideas so I asked forgiveness and told Satan to back off. God has the victory.

From that time on we have had an amazing sense of God's peace and presence. We are being covered by the prayers of family and friends, in particular my colleagues from CRE (Christian Religious Education teachers).

> There are no victims in the family of Christ. Understand that whatever happened to you – or will yet happen – is raw material for God to bless you and teach you something vital to the increase of your own blessing and development of your maturity. Nothing that happens to me can hurt me, unless I choose a wrong response, for it is my own responses that will leave me either better or bitter about life. What I am becoming, not what I am achieving, is what I take into eternity. (Source unknown)

Friday 18 June 2010

Graeme – Knowing that Shirley was likely to be out of theatre and back in the recovery room, I had been nervously lurking outside, waiting to hear, first and foremost, that she had come through the surgery safely and, secondly, that the operation had been successful. Amazingly, just minutes later Shirley was aware of her surroundings and, true to form, able to summon up a reassuring smile when she saw my anxious face.

Although the operation went well, we were disappointed to find the cancer had spread to the lymph nodes and several had been removed. The extent of future treatment depended on the results of the biopsy of these lymph nodes, which would take about a week. We had been mentally prepared for a short break and then a month of radiation, but the prospect of additional medical intervention put us back into the realm of ambiguity and with it came a degree of trepidation. It is always the step into the unknown that takes the greatest strength and faith.

Originally Shirley was going to be discharged the next morning, but with the discovery of additional cancer cells, we had to wait for the surgeon to make the final decision. Little did I know that this was a glimpse into a future where I was continuously left feeling frustrated. I could do nothing more than sit back and pray while the course of my wife's journey was being determined by a bunch of people in white coats.

Tuesday 22 June 2010

Shirley ~ Thanks, we are sure, to so many people praying for us, we all feel an enormous peace which allows life to continue around here as 'normal'. Normality, of course, hiccups at the point where I see antibiotics, anti-inflammatories, painkillers and other medical paraphernalia sitting on the kitchen bench. Am having quite a bit of discomfort and there is still a lot of swelling, so the 'crater' formed by the partial removal surgery has yet to be revealed.

We are waiting for a report on the dissection of the cancer lump and all the axillary lymph nodes that were removed – then we will hear the plan of action based on those findings. Meantime we feel compelled to ask God to surprise us all with a wonderful miracle. 'If you don't ask you don't get'. But we also know that:

All the days ordained for me were written in your book before one of them came to be. (Psalm 139:16)

God has not been surprised by this and has every day in His plan.

Yes, we want no more and no less than God's best, so we totally trust that He is in all that is going on, even if a physical miracle doesn't take place. Because God is doing amazing things in our family, there is far more to this whole situation than just finding a malignant lump. So we continue to be grateful to Him that we can rest easy in the confidence He is giving us.

Friday 25 June 2010

Graeme – About this time, many of our friends sent (together with the numerous cards and bouquets of flowers) books about people who had (one way or another) miraculously survived cancer (this usually involved some type of special diet). Others made suggestions about life-changing habits (such as exercise and stress management). Although we had discussed other possible avenues, as a nurse Shirley was most comfortable with the traditional approach to medicine. But, as always, she wanted to keep an open mind, and in this particular instance she was prepared to give anything a go.

So began a regime of daily walks, and rationalisation and prioritisation of necessary tasks, and out came the juicer. For a while we were subjected to some weird and wonderful concoctions (which, if nothing else, kept us regular) and so much raw food that we never wanted to see another carrot. Shirley was a great cook, so although we went along with the new diet, we were all secretly hoping it was only a phase. Thankfully, it didn't last long and we breathed a sigh of relief when the old cookbooks came back out.

Shirley ~ News isn't always what we would choose for ourselves, but we continue to know God is good and accept that He is completely in control. Unfortunately it was discovered that the original lump had spread further into the breast, an unanticipated setback as it had not been detected on the ultrasound. So although the surgeon took away a large margin of surrounding tissue last week, more needs to be removed. All of which means another visit to hospital for that, plus insertion of a catheter into the carotid artery for chemotherapy, which will start in a few weeks. The specialist has labelled this an aggressive cancer, which isn't exactly confidence-building.

Monday and Tuesday this coming week I have been booked for a CT scan to do a thorough investigation, top to toe of all major organs and pelvis, to make sure that nothing has spread any further. Presuming the scan is reliable, we should have a clearer picture of whether the coming months of chemotherapy are prophylactic or treatment – a tad different to each other. A great piece of news is that the cancer responds well to Herceptin, so that drug will also be given. In answer to several queries: no, it isn't a hormonal cancer.

Each time we go for results, we just expect them to be good then pop goes another bubble. But between the tears, we are at peace and that is beyond amazing. We attribute this to all the prayers being said for us. Even sleep comes quite easily and that is a very specific answer to prayer. It is an interesting experience to be on the receiving end of treatments instead of being the nurse. I am so grateful to those medical staff with the ability to be empathetic and give out comforting vibes when I most need it. God helps me to keep getting back to His peace when anxiety threatens and often uses others as His vehicle.

Wednesday 30 June 2010

Graeme - We met with Shirley's oncologist in the early evening to hear the results of the scans. This was a day we had both anticipated with a mixture of positive belief that all would be well and an underlying apprehension. Before we left home, we prayed that we would accept God's will whatever the future course might be and gave thanks for the many blessings we had already experienced.

One source of sustenance we never took for granted was the support of people on our prayer group, and other caring individuals, who continually sent us meaningful passages of scripture or uplifting paragraphs from something they had read. A poignant one at this time was 1 Peter 5:10,

> And the God of all grace, who called you to his eternal glory in Christ, after you have suffered a little while, will himself restore you and make you strong, firm and steadfast.

Our entire family seemed to be in a state of turmoil. Michelle was in the process of having shoulder surgery and had just returned from a well-earned break to prepare for her third operation. We were all praying that this would finally allow her to be free of pain and able to move on. Richard had been through a stressful few weeks at a crucial stage in his university studies, and we encouraged him to take some time out and go mountain-biking with his friends. Meanwhile, our star patient was optimistically pinning her hopes on her next bout of surgery.

Shirley ~ God has been intervening in other areas of my life. I have found the strength to confront a psychological wound I have carried for most of my life and feel it is the beginning of another healing process. I believe that it was God's way of showing me that we can be healed on many different levels: emotional, physical, mental and spiritual, and that He, not I, decides where and how to make the healing. Meanwhile, we continue to proceed with medical technology and believe that God's perfect plan will be revealed at the right time.

Thursday 1 July 2010

Shirley ~ Many tears are being shed at the moment. I guess it's a good healthy release since things happened so suddenly during June and it seems I'm experiencing some delayed reaction – a bit of shock is setting in.

Yesterday we received the scan results and were delighted to hear they have been returned clear. We understand that the prognosis is good due to the fact that the cancer was caught early – once again we gave thanks to God for His protection. My oncologist presented us with a few options and added to our emotional upheaval with a blunt reality-check by pointing out that scans do not pick up minuscule stray cancer cells that may have already spread further into the body apart from the four identified axillary lymph nodes. We'd prefer to believe that hasn't happened. However, we have very intentionally assigned our case to the Great Physician and trust that God will give our doctors His wisdom.

So at this stage it looks like I will be starting chemotherapy treatment combined with Herceptin at the end of July. That should put many things on hold while my body has time to recover from the onslaught. The thought of hair loss makes me shudder – yet there are many who do it naturally and live quite comfortably with it – so I'll be joining those ranks, but hopefully disguised with a wig.

GOD'S GRACE is coming out on top in my reading:

> My grace (or my favour) is sufficient for you, for my power is made perfect in weakness. (2 Corinthians 12:9-10)

And this quote sent by a friend:

> We may never understand our pain, depression and discomfort. We may never know why. But we don't have to know why. Our God has already answered us: 'You've got my grace – and, my beloved child, that is all you need.' (David Wilkerson, source unknown)

Wow, God is good. So I'm wiping away those tears and going back to bed – to sleep.

Friday 2 July 2010

> But for you who revere my name the sun of righteousness will rise, with healing in its wings… (Malachi 4:2, NRSV)

> Let us draw near to God with a sincere heart and with the full assurance that faith brings... Let us hold unswervingly to the hope we profess, for he who promised is faithful. (Hebrews 10:22-23)

Graeme – Through our daily travails, small miracles regularly occurred that were easy to overlook in the grander scheme of things. So we made a conscious decision to seek out the comparatively infinitesimal details and let God take care of the bigger picture. In other words: to count our blessings.

Michelle came home after her successful shoulder surgery with her arm in a sling again – which she was not too happy about – but accepted it was a small inconvenience that could be tolerated for a few more weeks. Richard was feeling far less stressed, and now that his exams were over, he was confident that he had done well. And with a little help from my Heavenly Father, I was coping far better than I had anticipated.

Shirley had surgery about 8 a.m. in the morning, and after being offered the choice, opted to stay overnight in hospital, encouraged by the fact that it cost no extra and gave her the benefit of proper care and hopefully a better rest. The Southern Cross Hospital seems to work like a motel – you need to vacate by about 10 a.m. or you pay for another night.

She recovered much more quickly this time and was more alert – for which we thanked God. The surgeon said it all went well and she was happy – it was all good news. So the next stage would be physical healing and recuperation, prior to beginning chemotherapy towards the end of July. So far we had received a cocktail of no news, good news and bad news – a turbulent period in our lives as we came to terms with so many mixed blessings.

Tuesday 6 July 2010

Graeme – Initially I was reluctant to leave Shirley by herself and felt very selfish to be indulging in a favourite sport and holidaying while she was so ill. But she was adamant I should honour the plan I had made some time ago with my nephew and Richard to go down to the snow for a few days skiing. Michelle reminded me that she would be there for her mum and encouraged me to go. Later, I gave thanks to God for giving Shirley the wisdom to persuade me to take a break. It wasn't until I was in a different environment that I realised I had been shallow breathing for what seemed a very long time. Deep cleansing breaths, inhaling pristine mountain air, filled my mind and heart (and lungs of course) with renewed vigour.

I had time to reflect on the course of action we had decided on after extensive research – careful dissemination of all the available facts and much prayer for guidance. Ultimately we felt compelled to trust Shirley's oncologist and (in our hearts) place him under the supervision of the Great Physician. We certainly could not have faced the necessary choices with the same courage and determination on our own.

Given his not so delightful report that 'Mrs Dando has a poor prognosis cancer…' the oncologist had presented us with two main choices. One: the tried and true 18-week course of chemotherapy followed by at least 14 doses of Herceptin (each three weeks apart). Or two: a course of chemotherapy (six doses) over 18 weeks that would include Herceptin, allowing Shirley's body to have access to the drug's benefits early and its apparent enhanced effect when combined with the first three doses of chemotherapy.

This second regime was the result of a Finnish study that produced comparable outcomes to the longer course and reduced the possible side-effects of Herceptin. The oncologist explained that Herceptin was still a relatively new drug and, while it was having very positive results treating some cancers, aspects of its use were still subject to trials. Our options were presented very clearly, together with a recommendation to take the second shorter course. We both agreed that this was the better choice at this point and trusted God to intervene where needed.

Shirley ~ This crazy journey we have been embarked on since early June continues, yet we are immensely grateful for the peace of mind God has given us and trust in His healing power. It's like nothing else.

Before the redivac drain was removed 10 days after the first operation, large amounts of serous fluid kept flowing into the vacuum ball. When the drain was removed, the fluid kept accumulating under my armpit into a golf-ball-size lump – a seroma. A trip to the lymphoedema nurse, one needle inserted into totally numb tissue, and the lump was drained. This happened again the following week and then the problem seemed to resolve itself.

I am grateful for the support of the medical staff who, before my second partial mastectomy, gave me a small dose of 'happy juice' before I went into theatre – so my next memory was 'It's all over.' While under anaesthetic, a port-a-cath was also inserted into my jugular vein for the easier administration of chemotherapy. We are now waiting for the histology results from the extra breast tissue which was removed as a precaution – the previous generous removal proving barely adequate.

By coincidence, Michelle and I were in hospital together – she was having another round of surgery on her shoulder. We had some girlie fun together. We arranged for Richard to bring in his camera and take some photos of us both in our theatre gowns.

We looked like the before and after makeover for a woman's magazine: Michelle was post-op puffy-eyed and pale; and I was pre-op and wearing mascara. We drew some amused smiles from passing staff. For a while there it appeared to be a Dando takeover of the ward. We have been indulging in a few prescribed painkillers, no doubt aiding and abetting our fits of giggles over idiotic things, but our wounds are healing and pain diminishing. So it's all good.

However, to a degree, 2010 has been put on hold. As I may not be 100 percent reliable over the next few months, I am taking a short break. A Bible CRE teacher is very willingly reliefteaching my class for the rest of the year and we are praying for someone to do the same for my other Year 5 and 6 class as well. One of my classes was given the task of making cards for their decommissioned teacher. I actually didn't need another reason to let the tears flow but you can understand why they did when I read the messages: 'It's not an exciting day without you'; 'Your name's in the clouds because you are an angel'; 'God is looking over you'; 'It's a dull day without you, you make the sun shine'; 'Stars will glow and you will shine, you're brighter than Sirius, the shining star, I hope you get better and go very far'; 'I hope you get better soon and come back to our class'.

Friday 9 July 2010

Graeme ~ Shirley was very sociable and had a lot of supportive friends who stayed in constant touch and made a concerted effort to involve her in their social activities. She also appreciated the fact that they didn't treat her differently and were not awkward about the cancer issue. I would often come home in the evening to find her tired but itching to tell me some titbit of news and she would cheerfully bemoan the fact that she had indulged in too many calories after someone had turned up with goodies for morning or afternoon tea. Sometimes friends would visit on some other pretext and end up helping with household chores. And each contributed their own pearls of wisdom, sharing stories and personal experiences.

Shirley ~ My prayers have been answered regarding relief teachers for my classes. In all, six experienced CRE teachers have made themselves available – hey God, we only need one! Proof yet again that God is GOOD, that CRE is His work, and He owns 'the cattle on a thousand hills' (Psalm 50:10). Everyone is making it abundantly clear that the new arrangements are merely a holding pattern until I get well. Likewise, with the great team at Mainly Music – my present role is to just be available when I can and be willing to take a back seat. Not something I am usually known for but no doubt good for the soul.

Our saga continues but my wounds are healing well and in myself I'm feeling good. I have a lot of nerve pain discomfort in my left axilla and down the arm, but have been assured that much of that should resolve itself over the next 18 months as the injured nerves relearn their function. I'm coming to terms with the prospect of the whole hair loss and fatigue thing but admit to the fact that my tear ducts have had an enormous flush-out on many occasions recently. But the strange thing is that it is always short-lived and I'm then left feeling okay again in the knowledge that God will be there the whole way.

Tuesday 13 July 2010

Graeme ~ At long last we had some wonderfully good news to share. When I accompanied Shirley for her follow-up checks with her surgeon, the histology report had just arrived from the recent re-excision surgery of the breast wound. We were humbled to hear the miraculous words: 'No cancer was discovered in the further tissue removed.' Although we had prayed for healing and believed God would respond, I had nonetheless prepared myself for the possibility of bad news. I had erected barriers in my mind to protect myself, so it took a while for the full implication to sink in and to realise we had just been presented with evidence that our prayers had been heard.

Shirley – Can you imagine how it felt to hear those miraculous words 'NO CANCER WAS DISCOVERED IN THE FURTHER TISSUE REMOVED'. Thank you, Lord. Thank you, Lord! And thanks too, to all the wonderfully faithful people praying on our behalf. God continues to keep us close to Him and to assure us He is in control. We trust in His healing power.

Monday 26 July 2010

Shirley – It is often the little things that sustain me and more often than not it is a thoughtful action by Michelle. This text is just one of many:

> Thought you might like this – 'We may throw the dice, but the Lord determines how they fall.' (Proverbs 16:33, NLT)

The last week or two have been filled with oncologist, radiotherapy (me) and shoulder surgeon (Michelle) appointments as well as all the paraphernalia that goes with organising, transporting and simply managing to stay sane through it all. But I am so very grateful to have the energy and ability to do it – ordinary things tend to take extraordinary effort when your stamina is not 100 percent and it feels great being able to catch up on several activities and outstanding tasks.

So many wonderful people are praying on our behalf. We love the enthusiasm of those who are praying against hair loss (wonder if God will answer yes to that one?) and the negative effects of the chemotherapy on my body. When a friend was praying for me recently I saw a picture of Shadrach, Meshach and Abednego in the fiery furnace, unaffected by the heat and with God right there with them (Daniel 3). How amazing is our Heavenly Father, sending these constant assurances that He is always in control and with us.

Chemotherapy and Herceptin treatment commences on August 4. Each of the subsequent treatments (six in all) will be three weeks apart, which takes us into December. If my blood counts are too low a treatment may need to be delayed and, on a cautionary note, when they're low in the middle week I will be prone to picking up infections. So I will reluctantly keep away from my classroom activities.

At this stage, five weeks of radiotherapy (Monday to Friday) will follow the above in early 2011. I'll consider all the implications and discomforts of that much nearer the time. We believe it right to continue through all the prescribed treatment. Medical technology has improved incredibly, even in the last five years. By using CT scans the precision of administering the radiation can be very accurate, hopefully avoiding the chances of damaging other organs and bones.

I've also asked friends to pray that God will give me the right words to encourage others I will meet along the way who may be struggling through these treatments and not have my 'secret weapon'. There will undoubtedly be many opportunities to share God's love with fellow travellers along this perilous path.

Of course I've had some anxious moments (times like 3 a.m.) but keep reminding myself that while I am plagued with unanswerable questions about my future, what is unknown to me is known to God and He is going ahead. And there are so many encouraging words and meaningful expressions of hope that always appear whenever they are needed the most. A brave friend who has continual severe health issues recently wrote:

> Even though it's overwhelming sometimes when we are faced with these challenges the Lord allows us to endure, I also know that He is able to see us through and bring us into victory.

The words 'life' and 'victory' have been significant to us since the beginning of this journey.

Tuesday 3 August 2010

Shirley – This evening Graeme and I visited friends to share the power of communion with them – 'by his wounds we are healed' (Isaiah 53:5). As they talked about 'the valley of the shadow' I realised how this theme carried from the original shadow on the mammogram that started this furore.

> Even though I walk through the valley of the shadow of death, I will fear no evil, for you are with me; your rod and your staff they comfort me. (Psalm 23:4)

> Whoever dwells in the shelter of the Most High will rest in the shadow of the Almighty. (Psalm 91:1)

What a glowing testimony to the security of those who trust in God. I will have no fear of the shadow of death knowing that God will shelter me. Now that really is a meaningful message.

Tomorrow Graeme and I have an appointment at 11.30 a.m., then there will be a four-hour IV infusion during the afternoon. Apparently the first session is slower to ensure all goes smoothly. I woke up last night at 3 a.m. (seems it's becoming a habit) wondering what I was doing to my poor beleaguered body going through with all this. But we have had much confirmation that this is right, so I got over myself quickly (fortunately) and thanked the Lord that He is there every step of the way. Amazing how this equates to peace.

CHAPTER 2

Stark Reality

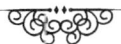

Wednesday 4 August 2010

Shirley – Stark reality! This is it – Dose One of chemotherapy today. Drugs: Taxotere and Herceptin. A very emotional moment as I was confronted with the enormity of what is happening.

Friday 6 August 2010

Shirley – Yay! Dose One over. I have been heavily drugged on steroids and strong anti-nauseous medication since the day before chemotherapy started. Weaned off the steroids this morning and left on the anti-nausea, much better than suffering without it all no doubt. When the oncology nurse rang to check me out the first day I commented that I felt really well. She replied: 'This is only day one you realise' – hinting of course that I was being premature in my optimism. Obviously not the usual reaction, but then she has not been dealing with someone under God's protection before.

Apart from all that, I am lacking in sleep majorly (only two to four hours each of the last three nights). I'm really tired. Apparently it is because of the high dose of steroids which will be the usual regime of medication around each of the subsequent doses of chemotherapy. During the second week of each cycle I will be on a strong dose of antibiotics to protect me while my blood count is very low.

Thursday 19 August 2010

Shirley ~ I am encouraged by so many emails and texts. To be part of a loving family as well as a Christian family and wider group of such neat friends is a privilege, nothing less. I constantly reflect on this love to keep me up when I am down. Now is the prime time, I think, to document the not-so-pleasant memories before they fade.

Copious amounts of medication certainly covered the first three to four days after treatment, where chemotherapy patients can be very sick. By day six my blood results were rock bottom (fascinating figures) and the best advice I received was to stay home, away from all the flu that is around at present.

Fatigue, itchy eyes, frequent loo visits and sore mouth seem to be the main events. The second week was unpleasant but all in all I can't complain. The whole process is an assault on the body. Selective hibernation is setting in; this is a lifestyle in itself but fortunately only temporary. Hey, I'm now better prepared to manage the next round. And truthfully, staying home is all I've felt like apart from my big day out for a blood test and Pink Pilates.

Pink Pilates is a trust set up by the NZ Breast Cancer Foundation. It offers a subsidised specialised physiotherapy treatment and stretching techniques which have given me a range of movement (in my left arm and shoulder after axillary node removal) that I thought would be very difficult to regain. Yes, I have been pushed way past my comfort zone and I am very grateful for that as it has alleviated a lot of nerve pain as well.

For four days last week my scalp was sooooooo itchy and my hair was so brittle and dry I was ready to forget my fear of losing it and tear it out myself. Thought that was it – falling out after the first dose, as the oncologist had said it would. Then just like a shampoo advertisement it became silky and soft again. I would love to keep it but I just told the Lord it was up to Him. Then last Tuesday while Graeme and I were reading an email which said: 'Wonderful that you haven't lost your hair,' I instinctively touched my head and a large tuft of my lovely tresses came away in my hand. Since then there's been increasing amounts.

Yes, tears (probably disappointment if I am honest – didn't really believe it would happen) even though I thought I had accepted the likelihood of losing it (and Graeme says he loves me anyway). I am still grateful to those who have been inspired to pray and feel I have let them down. But sometimes God says no, and that too is okay. Now it's actually happened I am more at peace and feel that it may be a way of identifying with others going through chemotherapy and similar disfigurements. Who knows? Only He does. That wig Michelle and I chose is on standby and gives me quite a chic new look.

Recently I've been reading and hearing several references to angels in the Bible and coincidently received a card with the same theme: 'The invisible host' that surround us as believers, ready to intervene on our behalf. Quite amazing how God protects us. When Shadrach, Meshach and Abednego were put in the fiery furnace instead of crying and whining about it, they spoke out words of faith – 'our God is able to save us…' (Daniel 3:17). At times I have got caught up thinking about my symptoms rather than keeping focus where it should be. I just love reminders like this – helps me get back on track.

After Dose Two next Wednesday 25th (plus three weeks) a

third of the treatment will be over. Does that sound like a countdown to Christmas? Feels like it – I'm like a kid counting sleeps.

This week finishes a run of tests and assignment deadlines for Michelle and Richard, then mid-semester holidays (a euphemism for more assignments). They are both stressed to the max and despite all evidence to the contrary are worried that they could fail or be presented with something they have not swotted for. I am determined to spend quality time with them and be there when they need me.

Wednesday 25 August 2010

Shirley ~ Dose Two of chemotherapy today. Drugs: Taxotere and Herceptin. Enough said.

Wednesday 1 September 2010

Shirley ~ Last night I simply couldn't go to sleep. My mind would not turn off and rattled around completely out of control. Since I was having no joy unaided, at around 12 p.m. I decided I needed a little help from my friends (of the pharmaceutical variety) and took a sleeping pill. By 2 a.m. I was still wide awake and antsy. So I went into the lounge and set myself up on Facebook. Completely unexpected, at some undetermined hour but right on cue, one of my oldest friends turned up.

Obviously I was so drugged I was almost incoherent and to an outsider would have appeared inebriated. Next morning when I read through the gobbledegook I had written, I cringed with embarrassment before seeing the funny side of it and laughed. Then as I considered what had transpired I realised that yet again I had been granted a small miracle. I was reminded that God never sleeps, He is ever vigilant and constant. He misses nothing: sees all, hears all, and interacts with us in a myriad of different ways – often using other people as a proxy to communicate with us.

In my (very late) hour of need, the person He sent to ease my concerns was also a nurse. I confessed that I had been struggling for nearly five days with a very sore throat and racing heart and was worried that it might be a side effect of Herceptin which can cause myocardial dysfunction. She talked me through it, reassuring me and putting my befuddled mind totally at ease. My double blessing was that it was all in writing and there in the morning for me to read over again.

Sunday 5 September 2010

Shirley – Not a good day. My sore throat is still hanging around after nine days, and although it hasn't developed into anything, it wakes me every night. Also have a painful spot, which I've mostly ignored, above the right breast where the port-a-cath is inserted. In my half-awake state during the night I convinced myself that the cancer must have spread to my throat, and had visions of having a tracheotomy and not being able to speak. Just the thought of how much more major this next surgery would be than what I have already gone through was enough to chill me. I leapt out of bed, googled 'cancer of the throat' and studied the symptoms. If I had felt bad before I was now beside myself with terror.

As if that wasn't enough, I also decided that the painful spot above my left breast was indicative of cancer spreading to a lymph node. Seemed so logical – I've already had four axillary nodes removed and radiation treatment will include the upper chest nodes but they haven't been checked yet.

Where has my peace gone? I feel really fragmented and it is quite a shock as it's my first absolute anxiety attack since the very beginning of this crazy journey. I was starting to panic when thankfully I remembered to take some deep breaths.

Today is Father's Day and I did want to go to church for Graeme. However he (rightly) mentioned that my white blood cells are still low and I shouldn't risk being with so many other people (and possible exposure to infections). Hate feeling so restricted, but okay, I'll be good and stay home and get into an absorbing book.

And via the book, God spoke His peace back into my soul:

But he [Jesus] was pierced for our transgressions, he was crushed for [my] iniquities; the punishment that brought us peace was upon him, and by his wounds we are healed. (Isaiah 53:5)

For God has not given us a spirit of fear, but of power and of love and of a sound mind. (2 Timothy 1:7 NKJV)

So whenever the old fear crept back in, especially while trying to sleep Sunday night, I repeatedly claimed a 'sound mind' and thanked God for His power.

Graeme ~ Quite frankly I don't remember Shirley ever uttering a negative word and she pulled herself up sharply if she found herself complaining – even in moments when a saint would have complained. But we certainly understood the power of positive thinking and, no matter what the circumstances, used only words of praise when speaking to God.

Shirley was ever vigilant when it came to preserving her relationship with God and often found ways to challenge herself. A passage she read to me from one of her favourite devotional books led to a discussion about the strength and conviction of our faith. We talked about the need to monitor our thoughts as well as verbal language and remove any negativity from our vocabulary. Unless we were both diligent in doing this it could be counterproductive to all the positive messages God was sending her.

Wednesday 8 September 2010

Shirley – Gathered my courage, confronted my fears and made an appointment with my doctor. She checked out my throat and said it was a throat ulcer similar to the mouth ones which can occur during chemotherapy (which, thank you God, I haven't had). And the painful spot above left breast turned out to be caused by tightness in the large muscle across this area. I drove home crying my eyes out with absolute relief.

Next day I visited the physiotherapist at Pink Pilates. She worked on the offending muscle and relieved the tension. Paradoxically the axillary muscles that had been relaxed at earlier sessions had sent another set of muscles into spasm. Thank you Lord once again for putting things right.

We continue to thank and praise God for His healing in my body and protection during chemotherapy. The white blood cell count, and other symptoms, are improving with the end of the Round Two cycle. Tomorrow I start taking steroids again as preparation for the third dose of chemotherapy on Wednesday.

Monday 13 September 2010

Graeme ~ Over the previous few months many of our friends had asked probing, thought-provoking questions about how our experiences were affecting our faith; as well as more specific queries about the medical side-effects. On the first point, there is no doubting the fact that this trial by fire had caused our faith to become even stronger. Other questions prompted a lot of soul searching and I had many lengthy discussions.

Mostly I was asked how I was coping and how Michelle and Richard were reacting to our family misfortune. I will attempt to answer the tricky first part of that question later (which may in itself be an answer – ignore it and hope it will go away, or simple denial). As to our children, both Michelle and Richard are compassionate and caring and had a very close loving relationship with their mother. As a parent, watching the mature way in which they put their own needs aside in order to protect Shirley and prevent her worrying about them was very rewarding. But then, we were being led by the finest example: in her day-to-day demeanour, Shirley was pragmatic about her illness and stoic about all those invasive treatments. We could do no less than accede to her wishes and treat her as the victorious person she was – Shirley never saw herself as a victim.

When it comes to the more personal experiences of this diabolical illness, Shirley probably put it much better than I could in one of her email newsletters, so I'll refer to that epistle:

Shirley ~ It's interesting how each of us react to challenges in our lives. I usually manage to put on a good public face and present a calm 'having it all together' front. As this whole process has been, and continues to be, a series of medically predicted stages, I've developed a way of coping by only wanting to be fully informed about my current stage. I have handled it better by being vague (basic info only) about details of future episodes and will face them when necessary. If people want to share more I may even suggest, 'I don't want to know thanks.' No offence meant.

Am I feeling afraid and overwhelmed? The first few days after the initial cone biopsy I was petrified. It was unreal. Yes I trusted God was with me, I had no doubt about that, but my situation and the word 'cancer' made me feel sick to the gut. But a short time later both Graeme and I were filled with the knowledge that God is steering our path and we can have HOPE and assurance for a great outcome. We trust Him for LIFE in abundance.

From that time God gave us a deep sustaining PEACE. However, there have still been many times during the last three months when I have been completely paralysed by fear at the realisation of what I am facing. That's where therapeutic tears find an outlet – sudden and quick, then I can move on. Last weekend when I convinced myself the cancer had spread and was thankfully proved wrong, I lost that peace majorly. As a Christian I recognise it as a spiritual attack on the peace that God has given me. Next time hopefully I will be better prepared for similar fears and press into His strength and Word.

Symptoms, you ask? Really I have been blessed with a reasonably okay time and I know God is protecting me. It can't get better than that. The severity of symptoms varies according to which chemicals are given, but so far I have only felt nausea as heavy medication prevents anything more. To list the worst: aggravated bowel is a pain; poor stamina and being tired is chronic; heavy drooping eyes; difficulty sleeping during high steroid times; throat ulcer; and thumping heart. Oh, and yes, the hair.

Wednesday 15 September 2010

Shirley – The Cancer Society has a Look Good Feel Better workshop. Last week I attended – an amazing volunteer works with each patient doing make-up and face massages. A bonus was being given all the make-up at the end. It turned out to be a fun experience. At the start, however, I was suddenly struck with the reality that I was one of the hairless wonders sitting in the group, not one of the team helping them. My emotions are pretty raw at times like that. It's an interesting little journey – many lessons in humility and accepting that I am no longer the one in control.

And yes, it happened! Stepped out of the car face first into a gust of wind and my wig flew off. Fortunately I had a small skull cap under it that time. Lesson learnt – will know to watch that pesky wind in future.

We have many scheduled events over the coming weekends and (somewhat reluctantly) I accept that I'm not able to commit myself in advance. Graeme will go to what he needs to attend while I get in some more reading and enjoy my own company. A no-brainer really as I have no intention of risking infection and being subjected to the inconvenience of another hospital stay.

Wednesday 15 September 2010

Shirley – Third dose of chemotherapy today. Drugs: Taxotere and Herceptin. No comment.

Friday 24 September 2010

Shirley – Yesterday an arborist pruned the titoki trees on our driveway. He very skilfully removed the large tall branches that had been hitting against the roof tiles and spouting during high winds; he cut off all the dead branches and twigs; and then he ruthlessly pruned the tree back. Viewed from inside the house, the amputated branches are obvious but from the driveway plenty of attractive foliage acts as camouflage.

So it came as no surprise when this evening while we were at a friend's home for our usual Friday prayer time we were drawn to the scripture in John.

> I am the true vine, and my Father is the gardener. He cuts off every branch in me that bears no fruit, while every branch that does bear fruit he prunes so that it will be even more fruitful. (John 15:1-2)

When God prunes the dead or unfruitful, unsightly, damaging branches from our lives it reveals abundant new spiritual growth. He does it expertly, lovingly, beautifully. Perhaps this is a good analogy for what is happening to me.

Sunday 26 September 2010

Shirley ~ God is a God of second chances. Tonight we marvelled, celebrated and were extremely thankful. Graeme and I realised it was just over three months since the first surgery. At that time we were told it was a simple, fairly well contained tumour and so long as we had surgery within three months that would be okay. As it was, I wanted it removed 'yesterday' so it was arranged very quickly. However, after surgery the surgeon was quite shocked when telling Graeme (while I was in recovery) that it was worse than she had expected. After histology results were presented at the end of June, we were told that if we had in fact waited longer the doctors would have been giving a very different story because of the invasive-type cancer and presence in the axillary lymph nodes. Soooooo… a second chance. What now Lord?

I also have a second chance to address my attitude towards challenging situations. I now know that when 'poisonous words' are spoken against me I can leave it to God to handle and that the truth will be revealed. And that even were they true, unkind words say more about the speaker than the one they are speaking about. My lesson in this is to love and forgive (meaning not to accept wrong behaviour but also not to condemn it) and put it behind me.

God has shown me that there are many types of healing and different ways to heal. Healing some of my emotional scars has been a side benefit to this experience I could never have anticipated and probably would not have had the courage to probe without His guidance. According to one school of thought, emotional scars can lead to physical manifestation (a state of dis-ease) if not expressed; and although I know I do not carry any repressed anger, I do believe it is healthy to examine old patterning and relationship issues. So I'm consciously releasing old hurts and exposing any lingering resentments and giving them over to God. I can't begin to tell you what a feeling of release this has been.

Monday 27 September 2010

Shirley ~ Got hit with a real wipeout late in the afternoon and wasn't good for much else the rest of the evening. Crashed into bed feeling hot and took my temperature – 37.7°C. The persistent four-and-a-half-week-long sore throat had become a cough. Bowels had been particularly unpleasant during the evening.

I didn't feel very well at all. I'm still on the 10-day course of antibiotics so decided to check my temperature in an hour (following instructions from oncology) and phone them if above 38°C (this would mean being admitted to Auckland Hospital for intravenous antibiotics). Graeme prayed against the sore throat and any infection and that the temperature would settle. Next temperature was 37.2°C. Thank you, Lord. Decided to bunk it in for the night.

Tuesday 28 September 2010

Shirley ~ Postponed Pink Pilates appointment as even though I had improved a bit I was still wiped out this morning. Graeme took me for my weekly blood test — somehow never quite so daunting when he is with me. In the afternoon I called oncology and described the previous evening's small drama only to be told in no uncertain terms that they would rather we had notified them immediately as I shouldn't still be having those symptoms. Oh well, it was worth getting a rap over the knuckles if it meant saving ourselves a trip to hospital.

Friday 1 October 2010

Shirley ~ Bowels have been too constant all week, some bleeding and very painful, enough to persuade me to make a visit to local GP. I have an anal fissure which explains a lot, and was prescribed suppositories. Let's hope that does the job quickly. I'm still pretty washed out and tired, taking much longer to come right this time; oncology nurse says it is the accumulation of chemicals in my system. However blood counts have come up well. Praise the Lord.

It pays to keep a sense of humour – this evening we had visitors and I was wearing my wig. As I opened the oven door a puff of hot air instantly frizzed a section of the front. Definitely not a look likely to be adopted by hair stylists.

Sunday 3 October 2010

Shirley ~ Yay! It's the half way celebration. What has been has gone. We are now halfway through chemotherapy and the roller coaster keeps going. This coming week I'll be having Dose Four, this time with a bunch of different chemicals. Believe it or not, Graeme is actually enjoying our appointments as we have caught up with Auckland friends going through a similar ordeal. Not the place of choice to rendezvous, but it is making the best of a situation.

This last round has been more drawn out and very tiring, and I'm still experiencing quite a few discomforts, plus acid reflux and fluid retention. At the time none of it is very pleasant (I'm becoming a master of the understatement) but I know there is nothing I can do but hang in there and I know it will pass. Meanwhile, I am grateful for every small victory along the way and continually count my blessings. Recent good news is that my blood counts quickly returned to normal after the steroid impact was diminished. Sleep has also come easier this time. God keeps His promise to provide strength and endurance.

Wednesday 6 October 2010

Shirley ~ Fourth dose of chemo today. Starting different drugs: Fluorouracil + Epirubicin + Cyclophosphamide. We were particularly aware of prayers on our behalf. It was like being lifted way above what was coming towards us. As a mere mortal, I knew I would find it impossible not to be extremely anxious about the different set of drugs and accompanying reactions; and I guess I could have given in to that anxiety if I'd chosen that mindset. But instead I thanked God for His amazing peace and that's how God kept it. I'm only on the equivalent of 40 mg of Prednisone for four days, so that is half the dosage I had last time, but the amount of anti-emetics has increased considerably in strength and amount. Apart from that I am good. Praise God.

Friday 15 October 2010

Shirley - We had a wonderful prayer time with a friend at our home. We all felt that this verse was pertinent to my situation:

> For the Lord gives wisdom; from his mouth come knowledge and understanding. He holds success [victory] in store for the upright, he is a shield to those whose walk is blameless, for he guards the course of the just and protects the way of his faithful ones. (Proverbs 2:6-8)

I had also been praying that God would protect me from the radiation burns and blisters during radiotherapy. And look what He gave me:

> When you pass through the waters, I will be with you; and when you pass through the rivers, they will not sweep over you. When you walk through the fire, you will not be burned; the flames will not set you ablaze. For I am the LORD your God, the Holy One of Israel, your Saviour… (Isaiah 43:2-3)

Monday 18 October 2010

Shirley – Reflecting on the after-effects of last week's chemo: by the first morning until Day Five a lot of fluid retention – visible around the ankles, fingers, mouth and a loaded feeling around the eyes. Day Six I suddenly lost a lot of fluid (i.e. weight) – quite weird.

Graeme – Despite being subjected to a roller-coaster ride on this trip through different stages of cancer treatment we had not been derailed. For that I attribute our inbuilt seat/safety-belt (being held close to God) and the knowledge that when we could no longer see our way forward, His light shone ahead to guide us. We were always given the strength to see the positives in any situation – otherwise it would have been all too easy to lose perspective.

We had been discussing the use of roller coasters as a metaphor for the previous months and found the following from the *Word for Today* daily devotional very apt:

> Have you noticed how some close their eyes, clench their teeth and wait for the ride to end, while up front the wide-eyed thrill-seekers relish every peak and plunge? They're all on the same trip, but their attitudes are entirely different. You can't always control what happens to you, but you can decide how you'll respond to it.

This is the verbal picture we were given post-surgery at Oncology to explain how easily and quickly invasive cancer spreads (also to justify to us medically why quite intensive cancer treatment is considered necessary in such cases): 'You see,' the oncologist said, 'at this point I would still give you only a 35 percent chance of surviving 10 years. With chemotherapy and radiotherapy it will bring you up to 50 percent. With Herceptin added to the equation it brings you up to about 75 percent.' Interesting statistics. This oncologist was well-researched and with a good reputation internationally. We were confident that God, as our Great Physician, had entrusted us to this doctor's care. As for healing, God is not deterred by statistics, neither did we need justification if Shirley was not healed on this earthly plane.

The whole experience of going through cancer treatment certainly brought the frailty of our lives into perspective and forced us to re-evaluate our priorities. Shirley, Richard, Michelle and I found that things we had thought important before were now of little consequence. We became far more considerate and sensitive to our individual needs. We were respectful of our different coping mechanisms and careful to give each other space while at the same time bonding more strongly as a family unit.

In our own ways, each of us did our very best to support Shirley, but the truth of the matter is that we couldn't walk in her shoes, and didn't know how she felt. So when a friend sent a letter sharing an insightful personal anecdote it resonated with Shirley's own philosophy and was very validating:

> Last year when I ran in the Auckland Marathon I learnt one or two things. The first was that when you're in the middle of the race it isn't helpful to think about what is ahead of you or even too much about what you've already been through. It's much better for your ability to persevere to stay in the moment, and just put one foot in front of the other. The second thing was that if the Spirit of God is in you (and He is) then He is also experiencing with you the unpleasant

physical sensations. I know that pain and sickness can make us feel very isolated at times – other people can help but they can't really share in what we're dealing with, but God is actually with us, feeling everything we feel. This is about as basic a revelation as you can get, but I love it.

So many fascinating experiences, such as this one, were shared; so many uplifting excerpts from gifted writers; and of course many, many wonderful and inspiring quotes of Scripture continued to flood our email on a daily basis. Shirley documented all her favourites and reflected back on them whenever she needed a boost.

Cancer is a word that puts fear into the most stalwart heart and many of our friends who had heard horror stories about cancer treatments were curious to hear Shirley's perspective. Knowing how forthright she was, they felt no hesitation in asking. In this instance, however, she was uncharacteristically reticent – she didn't want every conversation to be about her health or to impose too much gory detail. For the most part, she preferred to keep a positive spin on every experience and chose not to dwell on the negative aspects. Talking about it, she felt, fed the fear and she wanted to concentrate on the end of the road – not the bumps along the way. But at some point she decided to sit down and take stock of what she had been through and the miracle of surviving it all. This is how she put it:

Shirley ~ There are good days and there are not so good days. Some side affects linger and others pass quickly. I have my ups and I have my downs and the only constant is my knowledge that God is always at my side.

Now that I have completed Herceptin and Taxotere infusions,

things are generally tougher and could be potentially more difficult. But I'm hanging in there. Side effects vary from person to person depending on the strength and type of chemotherapy administered. At this point these are the ones causing me the most discomfort:

- Sore mouth and whole of throat – some ulcers. Irritation causes a persistent nuisance cough. Whoever invented very soft toothbrushes deserves a medal – anything else is out as it is too easy to cause bleeding around the gums while platelets are low. Baby food is looking good at the moment.
- Taste changes and appetite loss. I'm not a reliable food taster at present as anything I eat seems bitter or slightly unpleasant. But if I know from past experience that it is okay, then I eat it anyway in the interest of good nutrition. The spin-off from this is some much needed weight loss. The challenge of course will be to keep it off later. Don't watch this space.
- Tired. Oh so tired. Have slept and slept this time around – can't seem to get enough of it. Haven't even used sleeping pills.
- Blurred vision. This one is disappointing as I thought I'd get so much more reading and computer work done. But the impaired vision comes and goes so I work around it.
- Digestive tract. This is just a polite way of saying that regular episodes of everything travelling straight through at speed are less than entertaining and quite painful.

Over the weekend Graeme and I stayed at his mum's in Karaka. On the way we discovered why they have off-ramps on motorways and put Burger King close by. Graeme ran a red light rather than risk a bio-hazard fallout in his car (don't worry, it was a safe manoeuvre with no oncoming traffic).

An appointment with radiotherapy was so full of doom and gloom that the blahs set in. At the end I was informed that a lot of these things happen to only one percent of patients. That was another time when my peace was challenged, but again God heard me and lifted me out of it.

Have asked everyone to pray for all of the above. Every day we give these things to God and thank Him that He *is* working for good through this cancer treatment and is protecting me from a whole lot worse.

CHAPTER 3

Wonderful Partnership

Sunday 24 October 2010

> But because of his great love for us, God, who is rich in mercy, made us alive with Christ even when we were dead in transgressions – it is by grace you have been saved. And God raised us up with Christ and seated us with him in the heavenly realms in Christ Jesus... (Ephesians 2:4-6)

Shirley – Each day I affirm: 'I am united to the Lord and I have become one spirit with Him. Body, everywhere you go today… God goes. God is in you. The power of God is in you. The wisdom of God is in you. The VICTORY of God is in you.'

As a couple we have always felt that God was also a partner in our relationship and involved in everything we said and did, but at no time have we been more aware of His abiding presence. On this, the most tumultuous journey of our lives, God is so right in the middle and we have never before experienced such an enormous enveloping of His peace and grace.

Graeme – Our beautiful region had been putting on such a magnificent display of perfect summer weather that Shirley begrudged spending so much of it confined at home. So on

Saturday she dusted off her comfortable walking shoes and we drove down to Orewa for a stroll along the beach. To the casual observer we were just like all the other normal happy couples: strolling hand in hand, dodging the incoming tide, crunching on seashells, listening to the delighted squeals of children as they ran in and out of the water and soaking up the healing rays of the sun. Oblivion, sweet oblivion, to be momentarily removed from the unfolding drama that was our constant companion. It was a perfect start to our wedding anniversary, which we celebrated officially on Thursday 28th.

Wednesday 27 October 2010

Shirley ~ Had Dose Five of chemotherapy today. Here's hoping for an answer to all those prayers asking for the large syringes of chemicals that were infused into my body to do their designated job and eliminate any rogue cancer cells still hanging around.

I'm also praying that the main side effects I experienced last time will be less severe. The chemicals kill off healthy fast growing cells as well as the cancerous ones, so this is where temporary damage is done to nails, hair follicles, skin, digestive system, mucosa, bone marrow, and lessens the production of white blood cells, which causes a lowered resistance to infection. It's an interesting process.

During last week, an episode of high temperature and not feeling well coincided with the sudden drop of neutrophil (white blood cells). I almost managed to talk my way out of hospital by suggesting we pick up oral antibiotics instead. But meantime, blood results came through, and by 10 p.m. I was asked to go in, so Graeme and I trudged off to Auckland Hospital. An overnight stay until next afternoon was spent having countless blood tests, IV, antibiotics, and zero real sleep in a very busy ward. My discharge brought with it a strong invite not to hesitate to come again when needed. My behaviour will now be exemplary.

Wednesday 3 November 2010

Shirley ~ This is the verse God gave me when Mum had her first stroke at 58:

> But they that wait upon the Lord shall renew their strength; they shall mount up with wings as eagles; they shall run, and not be weary; and they shall walk, and not faint. (Isaiah 40:31 KJV)

At the time I felt confident that she would recover and move on in life. But when she died of a heart attack eighteen months later, God gave me such peace and the realisation that in fact the verse was fulfilled in her life, that she was healed – not here on earth but on the other side.

Saturday 6 November 2010

Shirley ~ Woke up this morning with my little skull cap half off. Went to the loo and checked out that skinhead look in the mirror. Sometimes I get a brief feeling of resentment, even a quick burst of anger that I have had to submit to this (they tell me it's a little like the grieving process). I do find it humiliating but, and this is the amazing thing, these feelings are always fleeting. The peace that flows to me is overwhelming. Graeme feels the same way and we are both surprised that we are able to have such an acceptance of all we are going through. Even down to my self-perceived laziness because I have to spend so much time just resting – I can't even read at times because of blurry vision or lack of concentration. I've taken on the saying, 'I just go with the flow.'

Graeme suggested we get away together somewhere up north for a few days after the last round of chemo has finished. We looked at the diary and saw only a seven-day space before radiotherapy starts. Being confronted with the reality of that next step in this journey hit me like a bomb. It released the floodgates and I dissolved into tears. Seems such a contradiction after my previous statement about peace, I know, but I sometimes feel as if grief and hope, fear and faith are opposite ends of a rope that is tying me in knots. But all it took was a warm comforting hug from Graeme to restore my equilibrium.

Graeme – It was at times like this I was overwhelmed with feelings of inadequacy. I felt hopeless and helpless, and frustrated that I was unable to take up Shirley's cross myself and carry it. All I could do was demonstrate (however feebly) that I was there, body and soul, every second of every day and would continue to do so no matter what.

Shirley had a close friendship with a deeply committed Christian woman named Julie who was also a cancer survivor. Because this friend lived overseas, their relationship was conducted primarily by email. Shirley always looked forward to the next message and valued the many insights and feedback which had been acquired through personal experience. It was also a great source of comfort to have someone who understood the spiritual and emotional whirlpool she had been plunged into. This is one of the first of many messages that Shirley kept:

Julie – I really do understand what you are experiencing, although every individual has their own story, of course. The effect of chemotherapy on every part of the body is devastating but I stand in awe of God who restores first your soul and then your body – that also happened with me. Going with the flow of the treatment can become all-encompassing but the 'afterward' is rewarding and purposeful as you sense being led 'beside still waters'. Trust has never been more appropriate to put into practice and it took me a while to be convinced that God believes in, promotes, acts out and wants healing – in each of us. I think my mind was the last to be restored and returning to work was quite entertaining at times.

It's good to know you are nearly finished with the chemo regime, and as my oncologist informed me, after that radiotherapy will seem a doddle. That was true for me and I hope it will be the same for you, despite all the dire warnings and side-effects.

Re-reading your email it's obvious you are filling your mind and soul with all the good things from the Lord, His word and encouragement. And Shirley, you have a wonderful husband (just like mine) to walk through this with you. You are blessed indeed.

Our weekly church group continue to pray for you to be completely healed. We hope you will feel the effects of all your friends around the world doing the same – your army of people praying – and that peace will establish itself in your heart and mind in the days ahead.

Wednesday 17 November 2010

Forget the former things; do not dwell on the past. See, I am doing a new thing! Now it springs up; do you not perceive it? I am making a way in the wilderness and streams in the wasteland. (Isaiah 43:18-19)

Shirley ~ All things (both good and bad) come to an end – today is the sixth and final chemo treatment. Guess I should be excited (Graeme is on my behalf – I have just the absolutely best husband), but I must confess that I am less than thrilled at the prospect of another loading of poisonous chemicals into my system and am finding it difficult to conjure up enthusiasm. But I just know that so many people are praying and I'm depending on their faith to carry me. It's a relief to pass on the baton occasionally.

We have been on such a learning curve that at times it feels as if we have gone to sleep and woken up on a different planet. Our hold on reality comes from the knowledge that God hears our prayers and we are thankful to each and every one who is taking the time to include us in theirs. This alien world we find ourselves in may be frightening but we have an all-knowing and powerful God to show us the way and defend us when we are weak.

I vaguely wondered why I wasn't given the tumour marker blood test result last time round (four weeks ago). Today's appointment with the oncologist revealed that the result had been 44 (normal <42 u/ml) and last week's result was 85. There was the hope it would drop by this round, but it has doubled instead. The explanation was that chemotherapy treatment often messes up the result and the test can be inaccurate.

So, a few tears to get over my disappointment and back on track reminding myself that God is in control and we trust Him. We aren't going to waste any time worrying.

Thursday 18 November 2010

Shirley – What a difference a day makes or, in this case, a good night's sleep. Woke feeling really refreshed. Then I destroyed my sense of well-being by mulling over the ghastly side effects I could expect within the next few days as the cocktail of poisons worked its way through my system. I was cataloguing the numerous ailments I had experienced after each previous chemo treatment when I suddenly realised that I had not registered the significance of the differences.

Listen up – this is it: The last round of poison (whoops – chemicals) zoomed through me without creating havoc on the way. No blistery, ulcery, tender, bleeding gums; no irritable throat; no uncomfortable bowel issues; in fact, apart from being very, very tired, there were no other significant symptoms. Wow – and I missed the point! I had already experienced a miracle.

So back to my other bed – our La-Z-Boy chair. 'Soooooo tired' continues to insist that I rest and allow this latest loading to run its course, then God willing I can move on.

Sunday 21 November 2010

Shirley – Woke up during the previous night having a mild panic attack – overwhelmed with fear that God had taken His peace away from me; that I have taken Him for granted; that people have stopped praying. I asked God to restore the peace and He did. Jesus said,

> Peace I leave with you; my peace I give you. I do not give to you as the world gives. Do not let your hearts be troubled and do not be afraid. (John 14:27)

> Never will I leave you; never will I forsake you. (Hebrews 13:5)

I continued to bolster myself the next day by listening to an inspiring talk by Tak Bhana and summarised it to impress relevant points into my psyche:

> 'All Scripture is God-breathed and is useful for teaching, rebuking, correcting and training in righteousness, so that the man of God may be thoroughly equipped for every good work.' (2 Timothy 3:16-17) Don't base your faith on another's experience. It needs to be totally based on God's Word, not what we think it says. All scripture is significant and powerful. 'Consequently faith comes from hearing the message, and the message is heard through the word of Christ.' (Romans 10:17) 'Now to him who is able to do immeasurably more than all we ask or imagine, according to his power that is at work in us…' (Ephesians 3:20) 'in all these things we are more than conquerors through him who loved us.' (Romans 8:37) 'Therefore I tell you, whatever you ask for in prayer, believe that you have received it, and it will be yours.' (Mark 11:24)

> Every prayer is answered: The Word of God is about answered prayer. No, yes, not yet, keep praying. God hears and answers. Great activity is dependent on great prayer: 'And we know that in all things God works for the good of those who love him…' (Romans 8:28)

God, I see you in this, no matter what my pain. Your Word says that.

If a trial gets you closer to God, it's worth it. If it makes us more like Jesus, it's worth it.

My best days are ahead of me, not behind: God will maximise all He has put into my life to use me for the outbreak of His power.

God is good, despite hardship: 'If we are thrown into the blazing furnace, the God we serve is able to save us from it, and He will rescue us from your hand… But even if He does not, we want you to know, O king, that we will not serve your gods or worship the image of gold you have set up.' (Daniel 3:17-18) No one is beyond the reach of the Gospel.

Wednesday 24 November 2010

Shirley – Just thinking this verse:

He himself bore our sins in his body on the cross, so that we might die to sins and live for righteousness; 'by his wounds you have been healed.' (1 Peter 2:24)

I saw a picture of Jesus being whipped. And I realised that He went through all of that so that I could be whole and healed. What amazing love!
Then I listened to another inspiring tape by Tak Bhana, Walking in Divine Healing and Health. Points which impacted me:

Deal with hindrances in our lives: Sometimes there are things we need to do first, like go forgive someone or say sorry. That doesn't mean we have to forgive others in order to earn God's grace. But we put ourselves in a better position to receive from the Master. A closer walk with God and inward changes are more important than physical healing. Generally when we are in trouble we get closer to God. Ask with passion and fervency: 'The prayer of a righteous man is powerful and effective.' (James 5:16) Health is God's will for us: 'Lord, if you are willing…' (Luke 5:12) 'Consequently, faith comes from hearing the message, and the message is heard through the word of Christ.' (Romans 10:17)

Tuesday 30 November 2010

Shirley ~ When I first found this passage I was blown away and saw it as confirmation that I wasn't going wacko; the voice in my head, the one I most relied on for answers whenever I was in trouble, was most assuredly God speaking to me:

> If ye abide in me, and my words abide in you, ye shall ask whatever you wish, and it shall be done unto you. (John 15:7 KJV)

Wednesday 1 December 2010

Shirley ~ I was contemplating how precious life is and stumbled (oh really!) on this:

> 'O God, you are my God, earnestly I seek you; my soul thirsts for you, in a dry and weary land where there is no water.' (Psalm 63:1) The continual 'stuff' our lives are made up of is the dry and weary land. Even a God-called ministry is dry

unless we seek Him earnestly. Nothing substitutes time spent delighting in God's presence, seeking and trusting Him with every area of my life. The whole perspective of life is challenging. 'Because your love (loving kindness) is better than life…' (Psalm 63:3) The way God loves me is more precious than life itself. Life is precious! So why is God's loving kindness better than life? God's love is eternal whereas earthly life is not. Everything else passes away, but the love of God, like His Word, resounds past the confines of this brief life. His love is far greater. (*Word for Today*)

Wednesday 8 December 2010

Shirley ~ It is an enormous relief to realise that we don't need to go through another chemotherapy cycle with its smorgasbord of surprises. Yay! As the discoloured and ridged fingernails continue to grow out and the tiredness lifts (slowly), the oncologist recommended that I start increasing exercise. Considering the general weakness of my legs and overall lack of body strength, working up to a better fitness level again, and more, sounds like good advice. Certainly the mind is willing; we will just have to see how the body responds.

This whole affair seems a marathon yet we are certainly getting through it more easily than some. God's peace and strength are so incredibly real – they have allowed me/us to accept bad news, disappointments, side effects, and other hiccups without major stress. It's as if others' prayers have kept going when I'm feeling a write-off and my 'chemo brain' hasn't been computing very well. Hard to explain, but it's like being wrapped in a comforter and cosseted. I am forever grateful to the many who are praying for us, but having said that, I am determined not to become dependent on exterior support but to rely on my own inner relationship with God. That is what is most important.

Last Monday I had an appointment with Radiotherapy at the Mercy Hospital for a CT scan, three tattoos and a planning session to set up for the future radiotherapy sessions starting 15 December. The 25 'blasts' of radiation go through to 25 January. Have made the appointments for 9 a.m. so that we can hopefully have some life outside of travelling into Auckland daily (we're exempt weekends and public holidays).

During October I was talking to God about this whole radiotherapy thing. I know I need to have it as part of the complete treatment plan, but (worst scenario) burns/blisters and other potential damage don't sound very appealing. Verses in Isaiah chapter 43 have previously had no special impact so I was pretty dumbfounded as I read verses 2-3:

> When you pass through the waters, I will be with you; and when you pass through the rivers, they will not sweep over you. When you walk through the fire you shall not be burned; the flames will not set you ablaze, for I am the LORD your God, the Holy One of Israel, your Saviour...

For the sceptics, trust me that this was no planned find. I received it as a direct answer to my praying. Amazing!

I was also grateful to some wonderful radiotherapy veterans who have supplied me with great advice for taking care of my skin to prevent too much damage around the target sites.

Updates on the tumour marker blood test results: Briefly, the normal is <42 u/ml. Mine had been well within normal limits until the end of September, then had increased to 85 by

November. Results just in this week showed a welcome decrease to 73. This will continue to be monitored three-weekly. With the chemicals decreasing in my body, it is to be expected that the tumour marker result should also decrease. And of course God is also in the equation.

Graeme ~ It sometimes felt as if we lived with a very large elephant sitting squarely in the middle of our lounge. The magnitude of the presence of cancer was potentially overpowering and intimidating, impossible to ignore; and yet, because it would not go away, it was easier to pretend it wasn't there and learn to conduct our lives around it. We both needed a break and I felt that Shirley would benefit from some time out so I booked us into the Scenic Hotel in the Bay of Islands for a four-day weekend.

The location lived up to its advertising and we had an idyllic view from our balcony overlooking an immaculately landscaped garden. We ditched the car and walked into Paihia, arriving just in time for the Christmas Parade. It was a reminder for me not to take the simple pleasures for granted: to walk arm in arm with an attractive woman and enjoy the easy conversation between two people who know each other well; to sit together with a mug of coffee in comfortable silence watching the sun go down; to reminisce about our past and make plans for our future. The break did us so much good that we resolved to do it more often.

Monday 13 December 2010

Shirley ~ On our way home after our brilliant break we stopped for lunch with friends at Onerahi and then again for coffee at Wellsford. As I getting back into the car (mentally admonishing myself for spoiling this lovely day with negative thoughts about

Peace in the Storm

the radiotherapy being imposed on me) I noticed a man with a leg amputation. I was immediately struck with the thought that this man's disability was permanent – not something that could be repaired with treatment. It made me rethink my own situation and be thankful that the coming 25 days of radiation had an 'end by' date.

Monday 27 December 2010

Shirley ~ We delight in the fact that God IS faithful. He showed His amazing love by sending Jesus to us, then allowing Him to die for our salvation and to free us from our sins. We all know, and will have experienced to varying degrees, that in this life we will endure pain – physically and emotionally – but God promises, 'Never will I leave you; never will I forsake you' (Hebrews 13:5) When we trust and believe in Him we have hope for the future regardless of the circumstances. We are so grateful to Him.

Great progress – eight radiotherapies down – 17 to go. Although there is no sensation during radiation exposure (like an x-ray), some discomfort is starting to kick in. Consistent skin care also seems to be a key factor. A vertigo problem associated with past chiropractic manipulation is an ongoing issue with positioning for the therapy but, praise the Lord, the only feeling has been some giddiness. I relax and focus on 'Be still, and know that I am God' (Psalm 46:10 KJV) during the short time of treatment, and ask God to protect bones and organs that are also in the path of the radiation beam.

Surprising how, increasingly, energy is returning. After five months of crazy fatigue it is great being able to walk up stairs or go for a decent walk without shortness of breath and that dragging tiredness. For this I am very grateful and often ponder on the fact that things I took totally for granted before are a source of constant wonder now that I am able to do them again. Nonetheless I am prepared for the fact that radiotherapy will bring its own tiredness as the body works on healing itself and restoring normal cells, so I'm sticking with this laid-back, go with the flow philosophy which seems to be the best way.

An updated tumour marker blood test result won't be available until next week. Here we go again waiting and wondering and attempting to put it on the back shelf and focus on other priorities. After all, we know God is in control and there is nothing we can do but surrender. Praise God we can go into 2011 knowing He is our source of comfort, wisdom and strength.

Wednesday 5 January 2011

> One thing I ask from the LORD, this only do I seek: that I may dwell in the house of the LORD all the days of my life, to gaze on the beauty of the LORD and to seek him in his temple. (Psalm 27:4)

Shirley – This speaks to me about what I believe God has been showing me over recent months – to seek Him more and more, to delight in Him. I don't want to lose the closeness to Him that I have come to experience. If this is the reward for my suffering then I would gladly pay the price.

Sunday 9 January 2011

Shirley – I'm 14 radiotherapy sessions down now, 11 to go. Although I have a couple more sensitive areas of damaged skin, I am trusting to get through this series relatively unscathed.

Monday 17 January 2011

Shirley ~ Twentieth dose of radiotherapy today. Although my skin is very red after each treatment, it is not burnt and broken, and I keep being told by radiotherapy staff how much worse I could be. So far so good equals copious aloe vera gel plus aqueous cream, plus a small amount of bulbinella plant where needed, plus God's protection. I have received many comments from specialist, radiotherapists and physiotherapist that my skin is looking good, overall, for this stage of treatment. Praise the Lord.

Thursday 20 January 2011

Shirley ~ Appointment today with radiation specialist. I am being given a total of 50 gray of radiation over 25 doses, in fractions of two gray. She said this is standard treatment for Grade Three breast cancer. I am managing to focus on the language rather than the content and somehow it seems less personal.

Friday 21 January 2011

Shirley ~ One thing that continues to astound me (although of course it shouldn't) is that, whenever I need it, the right person will appear, an email will arrive, the phone will ring or I will randomly pick up a book and it will fall open at a relevant page. Then I found this:

> God speaks to us in scripture, and through our inner voice but he also speaks to us through a conspiracy of accidents.
> (George Santayana, source unknown)

The 'conspiracies' often come in the form of the right word at the right moment from thoughtful friends. I am always impressed by the ability of my friends to find the appropriate quote or to express the exact sentiment and often put into words something I have been contemplating. Some of my recent favourites:

> Praise God is all I can say. That verse from Isaiah 43 is totally amazing. What a comfort and a promise of protection. God will not let them sizzle you too long on the barbecue – just enough to burn out the bad guys. Hallelujah!

> It is true, when we go through the valley of the shadow of death we fear no evil… He is with us. Your valley is almost finishing… just keep going strong. When we are weak… He is strong.

> I remain confident of this: I will see the goodness of the LORD in the land of the living. Wait for the LORD; be strong and take heart and wait for the LORD. (Psalm 27:13-14)

Monday 24 January 2011

Shirley – Friday was twenty-fourth dose of radiotherapy out of the 25 daily treatments. 'Keep in there!' was waiting in my mailbox from my dear friend who knows all too well.

'She is mentally okay,' the receptionist was telling the radiotherapists. Pardon me? I was overhearing the tail end of a phone call about me as I arrived a tad late (motorway traffic). I couldn't help but query the 'mental' bit. 'Oh, I was referring to the fact that some people just don't turn up to complete their course of radiotherapy as it gets pretty tough near the end.'

Yes, I do agree with that. However, after I've been positioned on the table very precisely, the treatment itself is relatively short. Measurements to the millimetre are called out between staff. As the now familiar drone of the radiation treatment comes on, I can intentionally relax knowing I am safe in God's hands. And with only one or two telltale tears escaping.

And remember that volatile tumour marker blood test? Good news, the most recent result has brought the level back down to almost acceptable levels. The effect of chemotherapy was pretty potent – hard to imagine anything tough enough to withstand such onslaught.

We've had a great summer break, all things considered. Lots of long balmy days out enjoying beaches, walks, friends and all the wonderful things that 'normal' people do. Graeme, Michelle and Richard also took themselves off to walk the 19 kilometre Tongariro Crossing with friends (there was a small pang of envy as I would loved to have done it with them had I been in better health). And we are all looking forward with anticipation to see what exciting things the following year holds for us.

> Real happiness comes from the inside, from God's Spirit living in us. So it doesn't matter where my body lives or what my circumstances are, I can still be content. (Unknown)

Thursday 27 January 2011

Shirley ~ Yesterday a friend asked me if I was feeling stronger and able to enjoy the tail end of the summer with walks on the beach and other outings. In answering I was reminded yet again that my recovery has been amazing – although still really tired, I feel stronger by the day. I also took great delight in telling her how, despite dire warnings to the contrary, I had no blistering or cracking after radiation and my skin was healing nicely. The only small hiccup was one particularly bad night when I had stabbing pain in the area which had taken the brunt of the rays, but the pain quickly subsided after Graeme prayed for it. Praise the Lord!

> when you walk through the fire, you will not be burned…
> (Isaiah 43:2)

This is an interesting in-between time when I'm asking God, 'Do I step back into things at exactly the same place that I stepped out, or do you have a different plan for me?' I am open to new ideas and prepared to take on new challenges but I am also determined that it will be God's will not mine. So I'm attempting to be still and wait for His instruction.

Monday 7 February 2011

Shirley – I sometimes find it difficult being around those with secondary and terminal cancers now that I have been so blessed/spoilt and God is allowing me to move on and recover. On the one hand it is impossible not to rejoice at my own miracle, and on the other I feel guilty that I have been given this gift and they have not. I am inclined to ask, 'Why me, Lord?' I guess I shouldn't feel that way because I do understand that we all have our own journey and God treats us so uniquely in every situation in life. It is not for us to understand – He alone sees the bigger picture and knows the untold story.

CHAPTER 4

Quality Time

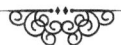

Sunday 3 April 2011

Shirley ~ Wow. TWO MONTHS. Two whole months of normality: of going to sleep at night with my head next to my beloved husband; waking to a day of interaction with my two precious children; sharing quality time with intimate family and friends; enjoying the fellowship of our extended family in Christ; and even feeling a sense of satisfaction from doing many of the mundane chores that make up our daily life. Two months! How could you put a value on that? And how can I ever show my gratitude to my beloved Father for granting me this time?

I freely admit I wanted to put any thought of illness out of my mind for a period while I adjusted back into our wonderful privileged lifestyle. But now I am feeling more than a little guilty for not responding to so many emails enquiring about the status of my health. So what follows is an overview of the last episode:

The final (twenty-fifth) radiotherapy was not relished in any way. I was meant to be celebrating 'the end' but in fact was dreading that last unwelcome zap. I asked staff for a protective barrier over skin that had become extremely red and painful, just this once, but no. Well, I survived without it. We have no doubt that awareness of effective skin care, and being covered by consistent faith-filled prayers, were all part of God's protection over my body throughout this treatment. Predicted deeper burns were apparently minimal and are being sorted out with the help of physiotherapy, and damaged skin healed relatively quickly.

At times I have wondered why I did not emerge totally unscathed by the effects of chemotherapy and radiotherapy. In that frame of mind I asked: did God not really answer my prayers and protect me? But those thoughts were quickly followed by the reminder that in every medical process I was constantly warned to expect far worse side effects than I ever experienced. Therefore the answer is 'Yes! He did protect me.' So I was left with the conclusion that without this personal experience I would not be in a position to relate, empathise and support those who did suffer badly.

To date, blood results have all returned to normal, hair is nearly two centimetres long (silvery greyish – ouch! my true colours are showing, but not for long), damaged fingernails growing out, and best of all I am almost running on all cylinders. The implanted porta-a-cath (very convenient during chemotherapy infusion) was surgically removed this last week. It is such an enormous relief to move on from all these things, but it looks as if some of the macabre jokes and innuendos we came up with to help us cope have become a permanent part of our family jargon. Our favourite being the 'Chemo Diet' – eat what you like and still lose weight; and sly remarks about homemade natural laxatives; not to mention windswept hairdos.

At the beginning of March I replied to an email:

Hawaii – now wouldn't that be a dream. It would be nice to just vanish into never-never land for a little while. I feel like I've been dumped off the end of the roller coaster and landed flat on my face. Multitasking makes me feel a bit overwhelmed and even a tad panicky. I do need to pace myself, whereas the 'old me' wants to step straight back into the shoes I had to step out of last June.

Looking back, we are incredibly grateful for God's 'peace that passes understanding' that we have experienced these last nine months. Whenever I became anxious, I asked God for His peace again and He always gave it. He is so faithful.

As Christians, our motivation is to give Him the glory in how we live the rest of our lives – our choices, actions and words. Only God knows the number of our days. We feel very blessed that I can move on and recover from these treatments. Follow-up will be every three months.

June 2011

Graeme – Feeling as if we had survived a shipwreck, Shirley and I were understandably loath to revisit any part of the previous twelve months. But with so many wonderful people standing by waiting to see the outcome of their loyal support and consistent prayers, it was important to give them some sort of closure. So I put pen to paper (so to speak) and sent out the following email:

> Last week was approximately a year since Shirley's cancer saga began. It ended when she completed her final radiotherapy and after the standard tests – x-ray, ultrasound and blood – came out clear. After so long and with so many different diagnoses producing outcomes ranging from exuberance to dejection, it seems inadequate to make such a simple bald statement: all results were clear. But since nothing we could

ever say would possibly express our immense gratitude to our loving Heavenly Father, we offer up our thanks and move on. It is pointless looking back, God has plans for our future and we trust Him.

Little did I know that we had merely completed phase one and there was worse (far worse) to come. The road ahead would test our faith and take us to our farthest limits. But for now we were resting and recuperating and rejoicing in a deepened relationship with our Lord.

'For I know the plans I have for you,' declares the Lord, 'plans to prosper you and not to harm you, plans to give you hope and a future.' (Jeremiah 29:11)

June 2011 – July 2012

Graeme - Shirley and I came to refer to the twelve months from June 2011 until July 2012 as 'The Gap Year'. It was crammed with wonderful family occasions that supplied us with a rich hoard of memories. A particularly memorable outing was in January 2012 when we went with our long-term friends and their children for a trek in the Waitakere Ranges. And although Shirley struggled to keep up, she just got on with it, determined not to hold us back.

During this time Michelle graduated from university and started her first job. We all celebrated her success and followed her progress with pride. It was also the year that Michelle and her boyfriend Dale formalised their long friendship and became engaged. We had of course been expecting this news, but nonetheless delighted in their happiness. Richard was also forging ahead and tackling all his university assignments with his usual aplomb. He was into his third year doing an engineering degree, and despite his casual acceptance of his achievements, we knew he was doing exceptionally well.

Shirley resumed a number of interests, including the Mainly Music programme for children and the annual Angel Tree collection raising money for prisoners to provide gifts for their children. Basically she was well – the only evidence of any problem was the need to deal with high levels of fluid retention, which was an ongoing issue she had been educated to manage. As a couple, we took a four-day trip to New Caledonia, after which Shirley graciously indulged my passion for American muscle cars when we attended the AmeriCARna car show in Taranaki.

Shirley and I lived very full and satisfying lives, and always gave thanks for our many blessings. Throughout both phases of our relationship with cancer we discussed the fact that neither of us had any regrets – no unaddressed issues; no unfulfilled dreams; no unkind word or deed unrepented; no failure to love and respect each other; and no real misdemeanours. We felt that we had followed as best we could both manmade laws and more importantly, God's laws. There was nothing we wanted to achieve or attain that, working together, we had been unable to accomplish to our mutual satisfaction.

So I look back now and kick myself that we didn't use this year to do the one major thing we had promised ourselves and intended doing for our sixtieth birthdays in 2012: an extended European trip. There was no real reason for us not to have done it, but that date came and passed, and we were still talking about doing it in the future. We were all lulled into a false sense of security thinking that Shirley was well and going to be with us forever.

We were in fact in a state of grace, filled with immense gratitude and enveloped in a deep sense of peace.

Shirley would often talk about being 'so tirrrrrred' and regularly took what she jokingly referred to as 'nana naps' when she needed to. But we had lived with 'tired' for so long that we accepted it as normal. The fact that 'tired' continued should, in hindsight, have provided some clue that the vile pestilence of cancer was also taking a break and regrouping for another onslaught. We were totally unprepared when the bombshell hit us. It was overwhelmingly devastating.

Friday 27 July 2012

Shirley ~ Felt a painless raised node on the left side of my neck. And to think that a year ago all I was concerned about was losing my hair.

Graeme ~ And with these unadulterated, simply stated words (recorded in a no-fuss manner in Shirley's journal) the next phase of our lives was determined.

Saturday 28 July 2012

Shirley ~ Woke up very relieved to see it was going to be a stunning day with not a cloud in the sky – a picture-perfect setting for Dale and Michelle's wedding. And I, the proud mother of the bride, looking and feeling fine. We had been anticipating this day for so long that it was hard to believe it was actually here, and Graeme and I were about to walk my beautiful daughter down the aisle to begin her new life as Mrs McCarter – I couldn't be prouder.

I am aware of a niggly cough that I've had for month or two. I am also aware that I get out of breath fairly easily, especially when I initially lie down in bed. Nothing to worry about, although it had crossed my mind maybe I should have a chest x-ray before going to Europe in two weeks' time.

Tuesday 31 July 2012

Shirley – At a reminder from Graeme that it would be no fun being sick in a foreign country, I finally made that visit to the doctors to check out swollen throat glands (which subsequently disappeared next day). I casually mentioned that 'by the way I've had this niggly cough for a month or so…' So the GP suggested a chest x-ray. This showed a partially collapsed lung with pleural effusion.

Wednesday 1 August 2012

Shirley – Dad's birthday today – 88 years old, isn't that impressive? Hope some of the genes were handed down to me. Thank you Lord for my dad who has always been there for me and is a constant source of old-fashioned commonsense sprinkled with humour.

Thinking about my health, I have that gut-sick feeling again with associated panic – just awful. Prayed asking God to give me His peace – I need that so much. He gave it instantly. He is a generous loving God.

Thursday 2 August 2012

Graeme – Some of my most enduring memories of Shirley were forged during this period when she demonstrated amazing courage. She always put on such a brave face, and although she had lost some weight, she looked well – exceptionally well. But she kept her health fears to herself and was not about to burden anyone else with tales of woe or self-pitying reminders of how ill she was. Her ability to state the facts relating to her prognosis and forthcoming treatments with such pragmatism was astounding, as the following journal entry demonstrates:

Shirley ~ Breast surgeon is now involved. Today had a CT scan. Had to drink a white mixture with barium first – not my favourite type of cocktail.

I refuse to curl up my toes. Many friends are praying. Wonderful prophecies are coming to us. God is good. Only He knows the number of our days.

> All the days ordained for me were written in your book before one of them came to be. (Psalm 139:16)

God holds the final card, but we'll fight this one with every bit of armoury we can dredge up.

But I also believe this whole experience has been for a reason we are as yet unable to fathom. Miracles come in many forms and, above all, my prayer would be that our children are drawn closer to Him through all of this and become very strong in their faith.

> Be strong and courageous. Do not be afraid [terrified]; do not be discouraged, for the LORD your God will be with you wherever you go. (Joshua 1:9)

Courage comes from trusting God, from believing what God

says despite circumstances. Discouragement comes from fear and disbelief, from listening to Satan's lies about what God is not going to do for you. We must rise up, despite our own limitations, in the Name of Jesus and the power of His Spirit and establish the power of His Kingdom of Heaven on earth. (Courage Comes from Faith, *Faith to Faith*, Kenneth and Gloria Copeland)

Friday 3 August 2012

Shirley – Graeme and I saw the breast surgeon today for results of the CT scan. The news: cancer seen scattered around the base of the lung with a moderate amount of pleural effusion; also multiple spots in the lumbar-thoracic vertebrae and pelvic ileum. Told in no uncertain terms that 'it definitely isn't okay.' Bearer of bad news that she was, nonetheless she was so supportive – really appreciate this caring lady.

We are going to the oncologist next week (Wednesday) for drainage of the lung. Both he and the current specialist insist that we should continue with our holiday plans since it is highly unlikely anything major will emerge within that time and medication will control what is happening at the moment. We are well covered with insurance so are seriously considering it and will probably still go.

We are all in this together, so we sat down and had a talk with Richard about the situation. Had Grandad (my father) over for the night to share with him and support him. Have chosen not to tell Michelle and Dale and interrupt their honeymoon. They need space together away from any pressures of life before settling into a new home and work again. I love my precious family sooooooooo very much.

Yet again, it's amazing how God's peace has kicked in – who knows, I may still be around for many years. God is sovereign and we have no doubt He can heal. We also know that He sees the big picture, and we only want His best for our family. It's all in His control.

> The LORD will fulfil his purpose for me; your steadfast love, O LORD, endures forever. (Psalm 138:8 NRSV)

Graeme ~ I am sure you can imagine how devastated we both were when another hand grenade was thrown at us. To stay with the metaphor, we wanted to leave the bomb where it had landed and pretend not to see it, so we wouldn't have to deal with it. We had fallen back into a comfortable rhythm of life where illness was no longer something that loomed over us and dominated every waking moment. We had been lulled into a false sense of security.

We were so ill-prepared that we almost felt like challenging the doctor and telling him he must have his records mixed up – these medical details couldn't be Shirley's. My emotions were in such turmoil that it took me some considerable time to come to grips with the situation and be able to consciously switch my mind back over into God's control. I clearly remember that I eventually found solace in the story of King Hezekiah as told in the Bible. He was ill and dying. He cried before God. God gave Him another 15 years. (2 Kings 20:1-6, Isaiah 38:1, 9-22)

Saturday 4 August 2012

Shirley ~ Graeme and I spent time this evening declaring God's truth and renouncing Satan's work in our lives and our family.

> See, I am setting before you today a blessing and a curse: the blessing if you obey the commands of the LORD your God that I am giving you today... (Deuteronomy 11:26-27)

Therefore I choose blessing instead of cursing and life instead of death.

> They were helped in fighting them, and God delivered the Hagrites and all their allies into their hands, because they cried out to him during the battle. He answered their prayers, because they trusted in him. (1 Chronicles 5:20)

> Be strong and courageous. Do not be afraid [terrified]; do not be discouraged, for the LORD your God will be with you wherever you go. (Joshua 1:9)

I will shake it off and rise up with courage!

> This is the confidence we have in approaching God: that if we ask anything according to his will, he hears us. And if we know that he hears us – whatever we ask – we know that we have what we asked of him. (1 John 5:14-15)

I will demonstrate my confidence and know that He will hear me.

Sunday 5 August 2012

Shirley – Graeme and I went to visit his mum for lunch so we could talk with her. Those closest to us feel so helpless and this whole process has been earth-shattering for them. We pray that in observing our faith and abiding peace with what is happening to us, they may achieve some measure of comfort also. So much of my comfort comes at the moment from my wonderful friend Julie, who seems to know just what to say and when to say it.

> I prayed that the blood of Jesus would flow with your blood and as it went through your body would heal every aspect of it. I very strongly heard the words 'do not be afraid'.

CHAPTER 5

Shattered Plans

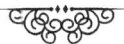

Monday 6 August 2012

Shirley – Graeme and I went to the oncologist for my appointment. There was no other way for him to say it – from now on its palliative treatment only, average life expectancy at this stage two and a half years, maybe five years. When he discovered that our holiday wasn't in a quiet relaxing resort but a full-on tightly packed trip including Switzerland, Italy, Greek Islands, Turkey and Dubai, he said: 'I wouldn't want to be hospitalised in Italy, definitely not in Greece, and absolutely not in Turkey.' At that point Graeme and I knew that we had to cancel our much anticipated, elaborately planned trip.

So now the plan is to have the fluid drained off the space around my lung this Friday at Auckland Hospital. Maybe a week or two later, a cardiothoracic surgeon will operate to bind the wall of the lung to my rib cage (pleurodesis). At some point later I will go on to chemotherapy – thank God this time only in tablet form and I won't lose my golden locks.

Graeme – At this point neither of us felt much like putting words down in writing; somehow their baldness made the situation seem surreal (as if it were just a story) and at the same time more poignant (forcing us to face our impotence). Shirley asked me to write our usual email and keep our prayer group informed. This is a segment of it:

> Essentially, they keep trying different drug treatments and when one stops working they try something else. The truth is they don't know how long a particular treatment will be effective and so it is a series of experiments. Shirley's life expectancy could be measured in years but the cancer will always be there, short of a miracle. They can't remove it medically and the oncologist described it as attempting to pick out grains of sand from her body.

To one of our friends I wrote:

> We are grateful for having more time together and will be sure to plan more carefully how we make use of it and savour each precious moment.

Tuesday 7 August 2012

Shirley ~ Friends have offered to come around and pray with us tonight. We intend to fast so have shared that decision with the many others who want to join us. We have reconnected with our wonderful prayer warriors and are much relieved to know we didn't wear them out last time. This is a very big exercise in humility.

Another couple also joined us this evening and anointed me with oil, lots of great prayers telling 'hairy legs' [Satan] where to go, in the name of Jesus. They prayed against fear and said that the words we speak have the power of life and death. The husband of one couple saw me in the Greek Islands (no, he didn't know that we should have been leaving for that part of the world in a few days' time). He also saw me holding a grandchild – that made me cry.

Wednesday 8 August 2012

Shirley – My Friday appointment was moved up to today. Arrived at Auckland Hospital before 9 a.m. and suggested that Graeme go back to work. Reunited with my lovely friendly staff. Little did I know the hideous day it would be. Got talking to a mother opposite who has a young daughter with a brain stem tumour and a lot of cancer in her family. She was soooo angry with God. She said that when she meets Him she knows what she will do to Him. I told her about the God I know, that He is kind and loving and explained that bad things in the world are happening because of man's bad choices. I asked her if she ever read the Bible – no. So I suggested she did and find out more about what God is really like. A short conversation, but hopefully some seeds planted.

The registrar in Acute Oncology prepared to do pleural drainage. Local anaesthetic given, then three attempts to tap the fluid. Not comfortable! She gave up, saying that I'd have to come back another day to have a radiologist do the procedure by ultrasound guidance. A friend texted me asking how it was going, I told her what was happening and she replied that she'd pray that the radiologist could do the procedure today. A few minutes later the registrar returned: 'This is unheard of,' she snapped. 'The radiologist has just had a cancellation and can take you soon.' She was clearly miffed.

So yet another needle inserted and 800 millilitres of fluid was removed from the pleural cavity. I was taken back to the ward with the drain still in. Unfortunately the fluid drained out very quickly and the pleural lining was irritated when the squashed/collapsed lung landed down on the drain, and I also started coughing. Or attempted to – but I couldn't take more than a shallow breath and the pain in my shoulders, left arm, chest and diaphragm was excruciating. Great attention-seeking behaviour, moaning, spluttering – I suddenly had five staff rush to my bedside to take my blood pressure and try to work out what was going on. The new registrar on duty noticed the amount of fluid drainage and suggested that 800 millilitres probably matched the predicted amount on ultrasound, so proceeded to remove the drain. Phew! Fifty percent of the pain was relieved immediately and all of it within an hour.

This afternoon Michelle and Dale returned from their idyllic honeymoon on the Gold Coast looking relaxed and so happy. We picked them up from their home in Milford and took them back with us to Orewa where we planned to share news of the last week. Michelle cried, 'No Mum! No! Who is going to look after you now that I'm not at home?' What a wonderful spontaneous response – that was so beautiful. Later they all fussed around together and organised dinner. My now extended family is even more amazing – I am so blessed.

Julie ~ This morning as I prayed for each of you I received this message: 'Because you have trusted me and have borne this news bravely I will bless you. I do not call on all my children to walk this pathway. Only the ones whom I trust. You have proven yourself trustworthy in the past and now are trusting me again. I want to take you deeper into me. As you share my brokenness on the cross you will also experience my resurrection power. Trust me in the darkness I will carry you through.' At that point I saw Him carrying you in His arms.

This passage then came to mind: Romans 8:17-30 – which speaks three times of suffering – 'if indeed we share in his sufferings in order that we may also share in his glory...' Verses 18 and 19 are incredible. They speak of our sufferings not being comparable to the glory which shall be revealed in us. It is those who have suffered who will then reveal God's glory and be transformed into 'sons of God' (totally transformed into Christ's likeness) and will usher in God's kingdom here on earth. What a high and holy privilege.

Initially I felt very down after receiving your email. I didn't want to say anything reflecting my personal shock at the news and I honestly was speechless. Now, though I realise the enormity of what you are facing in the natural realm, I have a different perspective in the spiritual realm. I believe you have both (Graeme too, because he is a co-sufferer) been chosen to be 'sons of God'.

Well goodnight my precious friend. I love you so much and wish I could take this cup from you, but as the Lord Himself said: 'Not my will but Thine be done.'

Thursday 9 August 2012

Shirley – A great combined family evening at Michelle and Dale's – wedding present opening and apple crumble. Good company (the best), fun and laughter, the excuse for celebration and my favourite food – lovely, lovely, lovely! I always thought I had the perfect family and it could get no better, but the addition of Dale has given us another dimension and our family keeps getting bigger and better.

Friday 10 August 2012

Shirley ~ Graeme's sixtieth birthday today – can't believe he has actually hit this landmark – he doesn't look a day older than he did on the day I married him. It's another great reason for a family get-together and celebration. And an excuse yet again for me to indulge in nostalgic memories of wonderful times spent together and the thousand and one ways I love and appreciate him. Thank you Lord for the most wonderful, loving and committed husband you could ever have given me.

The whole family went out to a favourite local Mexican restaurant for dinner. I would hate to ever take for granted the easy camaraderie that comes with people who have known each other for a long time and have a mutual history – we have so many 'in jokes' we could write a book. Afterwards we trotted back home to blow out the candles on a Black Forest cake. Purchased I'm afraid – nice but (everyone agrees) not up to the standard of the punchy flavour of the one I usually make each year. Just a temporary lapse in tradition.

> 'And hope does not disappoint us, because God has poured out his love into our hearts by the Holy Spirit, whom he has given us.' (Romans 5:5)
>
> In Jesus' name, I make a fresh and strong commitment today to live the life of love, to let the tenderness of God flow through me and heal the wounded hearts of those I meet. Father, teach me to love even when things go wrong. To be patient and kind, to overlook angry words. Teach me to talk in love, to lay gossip quietly aside and to take up words of grace instead.
>
> Lord, your Word says that your love is already inside me,

that it has been shed abroad in my heart. So today I resolve to remove every obstacle that would keep that love from flowing freely into the lives of others. I put resentments behind me and I forgive all those who've done me wrong. Cause me to increase and excel and overflow with your love. Cause me to be what the world needs most of all…a living example of love. Amen. (A Living Example of Love, *Faith to Faith*, Kenneth and Gloria Copeland)

Sunday 12 August 2012

Shirley ~ Graeme's old flatmates and Navigator buddies got together and organised a surprise birthday party for him last night. As close friends, they obviously knew how much he had needed to escape all this stress for a while. Such good company, lots of laughter, and great food. It was a much needed consolation for the trip we should have been embarking on today en route to Helsinki and Zurich.

This evening we went to a healing meeting. It was very low key which is great – God definitely given all the glory. Seriously I find it confusing because I want to believe God has healed as they claim. Does that mean I stop pursuing other treatments? If I continue, would that show lack of faith? Does it mean I must choose one way or the other? I value the opinion of others but am waiting on God's word – I know He will direct me in His own time.

Monday 13 August 2012

Shirley ~ Short of a miracle it doesn't look good. Is too unbearable to think about. It's the pain for my poor darling family.

The path automatically prescribed by doctors is well-worn and at this stage, medically speaking, it is like their last resort to try and control the invasive/aggressive cancer cells that withstood the hammering of a tough chemotherapy regime 18 months ago. I feel so strongly that God's healing touch is on me, that the LIFE I chose last time still applies today. He is building His kingdom and I believe He wants His people to suffer and be in various places to witness for Him. Only He knows and I trust Him. We need prayer that Graeme and I will know God's will when it comes to choosing treatments. The side effect of the chemotherapy tablets, although different from the previous IV infusion, sounds pretty debilitating and yuck.

Julie ~ My husband was praying for you yesterday and stopped and said, 'I believe Shirley will be healed. I do not believe it is God's time for her to die.' To set this in perspective he continued, 'If it be God's will.' For him to be so adamant is out of character. I was so blessed when he said that. Yes, you should believe with those who prayed at the healing meeting that you are healed. You thank the Lord for His healing. And you should have further prayer for healing. I do not believe that by continuing with medical treatment you are denying the healing that has or will take place. You take everything with thanks as a means of God's healing for you. But yes, you do need to be discerning and pray about each treatment, whether physical or spiritual, until you have God's peace about it first.

Tuesday 14 August 2012

Shirley ~ A day to reflect. Experiencing overwhelming numbness about my prognosis (horrible word). Looking to God and catching a glimpse that He has the big picture and is in control. Oh that is such a comfort.

Wednesday 15 August 2012

Shirley ~ I am feeling so sad about our Europe trip. From having a positive mind last evening, focusing on and believing in the power of prayer, my disappointment has dragged me down.

In the middle of the doldrums I received a text message from a friend inviting me to join her and six other women for coffee. Their energy was invigorating. Great fellowship, encouraging building up in the Lord – He knew I needed just that at that moment. Again mention was made of Shadrach, Meshach and Abednigo from Daniel.

> If we are thrown into the blazing furnace, the God we serve is able to deliver [save] us from it, and He will deliver [rescue] us... (Daniel 3:17)

Thursday 16 August 2012

Shirley ~ The hospice received a referral from the oncology specialist and called me today. It felt so devastatingly terminal. My response must have conveyed something of what I was thinking because they quickly assured me it was just to set up a meeting so they could tell me about the services they offer. They also pointed out that they aren't only there for people who are dying. Well-meaning as they were, it made me feel awful. It's unbelievable that this is happening to me. It's overwhelming getting my head around everything. I have cried torrents.

Blew my nose and decided to put that lot into the too hard

basket at present. So I have given myself a good talking-to and intend to get my thinking straight and keep it there.

Set your minds on things above... (Colossians 3:2)

Whatever is true, whatever is noble, whatever is right, whatever is pure, whatever is lovely, whatever is admirable – if anything is excellent or praiseworthy – think about such things. (Philippians 4:8)

Do not conform to the pattern of this world, but be transformed by the renewing of your mind. Then you will be able to test and approve what God's will is – his good, pleasing and perfect will. (Romans 12:2)

Whosoever cometh to me, and heareth my sayings, and doeth them, I will show you to whom he is like: he is like a man which built an house, and digged deep, and laid the foundation on a rock: and when the flood arose, the stream beat vehemently upon that house, and could not shake it: for it was founded upon a rock. (Luke 6:47-48 KJV)

CHAPTER 6

Reality of Faith

Friday 17 August 2012

Shirley – I woke up at 1 a.m. feeling restless. I'm in a real dilemma and questioning my own integrity. Some people think I should be saying 'I am healed.' Does this mean that if I am not healed I don't have enough faith? Then it seems like a double standard to me to pursue pleurodesis surgery, discuss treatments and visit the hospice.

To help clear my head I decided to write down my conclusions to keep me feeling right before the Lord:

- I totally believe that God has heard/is hearing our ongoing prayers for healing. Yes, He wants me whole. Cancer is not of Him. How He does that healing is up to Him. Our ways aren't always His ways.
- His healing can be a process, so I need to keep pursuing treatments confidently, knowing that God has touched me – but I don't know in what way. I simply trust Him. I don't need to continually tell everyone that I've been healed when there is no evidence. I will thank Him and say that God knows the very best for me, He knows the number of my days and I trust Him to work that out for me.

- So I keep thanking Him for healing, for the life I've had, and my life to come. I praise Him.
- I will go to the hospice introduction appointment on Monday confidently. They have services to support me along the way. They too can witness God's miracles in my life.

Having written my conclusions I felt much better and was sitting down with a cuppa when this reaffirming email arrived:

Julie ~ You are a Woman of Integrity. One thousand percent with you on your conclusions. Totally in line with what I wrote three days ago. God either heals you or He doesn't. He is not sitting up there measuring your faith to see if it is perfect enough for Him to dish out healing or not. And having already healed you, He will not retract it because you went ahead with other treatments. Like salvation, healing is a gift from God totally irrespective of the person and based on His amazing grace. On earth Jesus healed Jews and non-Jews alike (i.e. whether they were the chosen people or not). He DID reward faith, it is true, but He honoured faith as small as a mustard seed.

Claim your healing and thank Him for it. Live in an atmosphere of praise with music playing to keep doubts and lies from the enemy at bay. This is the biggest test you have ever faced and you are doing so valiantly and encouraging everyone around you, including myself, with your trust in God's goodness.

Wednesday 22 August 2012

Shirley ~ After visiting the physiotherapist today and showing her a painful mass above my left collar bone, she confirmed that it was glands rather than muscle. I have gained a lot of respect and appreciation for the wonderful support of the professionals I've had contact with over these last two years. So when I hear comments like: 'There is nothing more we could have done,' and 'You could say we have ever-monitored your progress,' I come away feeling incredibly sad. Sad about my possible lack of future here on earth; concern for all those praying who may become disillusioned and conclude, 'What's the point?' I think my crying could have filled a swimming pool this afternoon.

Two wonderful friends online to talk to – one lost her husband suddenly two years ago and knows the emotional pain we feel:

> It is natural to have those feelings and doubt. Keep looking up and don't focus on the logical conclusion.

Life Group tonight – study on Moses. It struck me that the only answer we can give faithful friends and family who are praying for my healing is:

> God said to Moses, 'I AM WHO I AM. This is what you are to say...' (Exodus 3:14)

And,

> The Lord will fulfil his purpose for me; your steadfast love, O LORD, endures forever. (Psalm 138:8 NRSV)

Checked my emails before calling it a night and, God bless her, yet another response to my deepest concerns:

Julie ~ I was acutely aware of the internal battle you are going through and want you to know that it is a normal thing to experience such grief and questioning. After talking to you I lay down and had a little talk to God. His reply was almost instantaneous and very profound. God's plan for you is HEALING on a lateral continuous plane that stretches into infinity. God sees our lives on a continuum that has no compartments for earth and heaven because He has conquered death for all time. So the answer to your wanting to know His will about healing you is this: God loves you intimately and desires your healing and wholeness. Whether it happens in the reality of 'now' and 'here' as we understand them, or on the other side of the veil, where there is no disease or pain and no weeping, is His secret and His mystery. But heal you He will. Therefore, it is honest and right to pursue healing and to claim it and leave the outworking of it to Him. It is also not being faithless to take what help medical science can offer, as it is surely inspired by the Creator to reduce human suffering.

As for your concern for those believing you will be healed and fasting and praying for you: you are doing us all a favour – giving us a reason to grasp the horns of the altar and thus come closer to the Master ourselves. Don't worry your pretty head about the time and energy expended on your behalf. You are ushering us into heaven's courts and we will all thank you for that in the long run. Also, it is our choice to believe and pray – besides, you are definitely worth fighting over. Praying for you and believing with you.

> Faith is being sure of what we hope for and certain of what we do not see. (Hebrews 11:1)

Sunday 26 August 2012

Shirley – We WILL keep hoping for healing 'this side of the veil'. Just hoping so much that healing is in this world. Graeme's picture of Hezekiah asking for more time and getting 15 years is very vivid in my mind. But the future's not mine to see and we trust totally in the One who does.

Received a phone call from a friend – she told me that she responded to the altar call at church today. She went forward to pray for my situation. And she is just one of many who have done similar things on my behalf – so many people are believing I will be healed and praying for me. God is doing amazing things in people's hearts. Praise the Lord. This is so humbling.

And thinking God helps those who help themselves, and nothing ventured, nothing gained, I decided it was time to check out other options and pay a visit to a naturopathic health store. So I trundled off on Saturday. Either the woman was a top-notch salesperson or I am extremely gullible as I left with coriander and tumeric medications and the assurance that it would improve my immune system. I also came out with enough nutritional information to sink a ship and the horrifying realisation that (according to my blood group type) I've been eating the wrong foods all my life. Well, that explains everything. Apparently a gluten-free, dairy-free, wheat and oat-free diet is an absolute essential for my type. Seems to me there's not much left to eat, but I will diligently sift through all of this and make a reasonable, sustainable, edible, sociable and achievable decision – probably in the time it takes to drop the lot in the nearest rubbish bin.

Tuesday 28 August 2012

Shirley – I need answers but no one seems in a hurry in this part of the world. Have decided that God must be delaying them. So tonight I googled possible side effects from pleurodesis. Put simply: it's awful. Quite obviously the procedure isn't done with longevity in mind. It appears to be a sort of quick fix to save you having to go through countless pleural cavity drainages and keep you going till you die. Language is soooo powerful and what I read was so graphic it set me off into a prolonged crying jag. My poor hubby and kids. God please save me from this.

I've since discovered that these are the extreme side-effects (not that it makes me feel any better) and that 90 percent of procedures are very effective.

Overcame my initial scientism and trialled the immune cleanser I got from the health shop – thought it couldn't make things any worse. Maybe not for me, but after a small 'return' by the coriander mixture, Graeme very unselfishly suggested I keep it for my own use. Did I mention that I had subjected him to the same cleansing process? Some of these concoctions were rather repulsive and I jokingly referred to them as a 'love potion' that I was taking to get better for Graeme. So that lot made it into the rubbish as well.

Reading the 'abiding' chapter in John this morning –

> If you remain in me and my words remain in you, ask whatever you wish, and it will be given you. (John 15:7)

At first glance it is seriously difficult to understand. The conclusion I keep coming to is that God is far more interested in the time I spend with Him than the time spent serving Him. It's always an ongoing challenge that I know so many others have also struggled with. He wants us to have a greater 'Mary' emphasis in our lives (the Mary/Martha balance – Luke 10:38-42). He wants us to WAIT and LISTEN to Him as well as read His Word and pray.

Thursday 30 August 2012

Shirley – Finally able to touch base with the oncologist. All my feeble reasons why they should delay doing a pleurodesis fell on deaf ears. 'Sooner the better,' he stated. 'The longer the lung is collapsed, the more difficulty it has inflating back to normal and there is a greater chance of complications.' Okay, that all sounds pretty convincing. Enormous grief yet again as I contemplate the fact that the operation seems radical in terms of future lung function. What if I live much longer than they predict? Wooah – am I actually having this discussion with myself?!

My heart is full of joy that God is speaking into our children's lives and using them to encourage us. Richard shared these verses with me this evening:

> Therefore I tell you, do not worry about your life, what you will eat or drink; or about your body, what you will wear. Is not life more important than food and the body more important than clothes? Look at the birds of the air; they do not sow or reap or store away in barns, and yet your Heavenly Father feeds them. Are you not much more valuable than they? Who of you by worrying can add a single hour to his life? And why do you worry about clothes? See how the lilies of the field grow. They do not labour or spin. Yet I tell you that not even Solomon in all his splendour was dressed like

one of these. If that is how God clothes the grass of the field, which is here today and tomorrow is thrown into the fire, will he not much more clothe you, O you of little faith? So do not worry, saying, 'What shall we eat?' or 'What shall we drink?' or 'What shall we wear?' For the pagans run after all these things, and your Heavenly Father knows that you need them. But seek first his kingdom and his righteousness, and all these things will be given to you as well. Therefore do not worry about tomorrow, for tomorrow will worry about itself. Each day has enough trouble of its own. (Matthew 6:25-34)

Friday 31 August 2012

A cheerful heart is good medicine, but a crushed spirit dries up the bones. (Proverbs 17:22)

Shirley ~ Supposed to have heard from Auckland Hospital today about the operation. Still no word. My only thought is that God is causing the delay and it must be for a reason.

A friend who visited me today shared an interesting incident from last week. She had been walking in Orewa and was approached by two ladies. They said that God had told them they should pray for someone regarding 'bones – specks on bones'. She went on to say:

We felt excited about this message and thought it may be directed at your healing. At the same time we are attempting not to put our own definition on things and to submit to God. We are learning and He is teaching. He has such a different way of seeing things than us. These are the words He gave us: 'Little marks / specks; not aligned; sadness / remorse;

communication; joy; mildew removal guaranteed; bones; bone marrow.'

They concluded by saying that they were keen to get together to pray for me about these things.

Tuesday 4 September 2012

'O Lord, see how my enemies persecute me! Have mercy and lift me up from the gates of death, that I may declare your praises in the gates of the Daughter of Zion and there rejoice in your salvation.' (Psalm 9:13-14)

David wasn't asking God to deliver him just so he could be free from the pain of suffering although I am sure there was a sincere desire to be free from it. David shows here another motivation – a deeper motivation. David wanted to be able to testify to others of God's goodness and salvation to him. This is a wonderful perspective. David knew that God was good. David knew that God was faithful. David knew that God could heal him. David knew that God could deliver him. And David wanted others to know God as he did and he wanted his life to be a testimony of what he knew of God.

So why do you want to be healed or delivered? Is it just so you can be free from discomfort… or is it so that you can further testify of God's goodness? (*Believing in You Daily Devotional*, Steve McCracken of David McCracken Ministries)

Shirley – I pray all of our lives are a testimony to the goodness, greatness and incredible love of our wonderful God.

Julie – This is just a little message to tell you that last night, as I was praying for Graeme, Michelle and Richard, the image I had of God taking care of them was the one from Luke 13:34 – the Lord as mother hen, gathering her chicks close under her wings.

Shirley ~ My reply: That is so beautiful. Thanks. Had a little cry over that one. God does know what He's doing in each of our lives – in fact He doesn't need to have YOU and ME for Him to fulfil His purposes in our family's lives. Now that's a revelation and so true. In fact we are so privileged that He has given them to us on loan and that He does use us. Can never take the blessing for granted.

Wednesday 5 September 2012

> Out of the overflow of the heart the mouth speaks. The good man brings good things out of the good stored up in him and the evil man brings evil things out of the evil stored up in him. (Matthew 12:34-35)

Shirley ~ Met today with the two ladies who shared the words they believed came from God (31 August) and their relevance to my life. We prayed forgiveness and God's love and truth into the situation, claiming freedom from this cancer and the spirit of death. They offered prayers that stated God will heal me now, in this life, and I believed it. It made so much sense. I was also in awe of a God who would prompt a stranger to intervene on His behalf.

Graeme and I went out to the church prayer meeting this evening. The theme was 'All things are possible with God'. The words of a song that we sang included, 'it's not how I feel, it's not what I see...' Okay, I can and want to accept that.

I had a call from the oncologist talking about this darn pleurodesis. I was left deliberating over the major question: If God has/is healing me, why would I agree to have this somewhat debilitating procedure done? It's all so confusing! If God wants me to die, why doesn't He just make it happen instead of letting me live in this double standard state? I said that I want God's best. What is that? Blind trust, again. I guess that's my answer.

Thursday 6 September 2012

Shirley – Didn't take any of my immune-building medicine this morning – thought, what's the point? Cried so much, especially when I read the passage below, I could so completely identify with how David felt. Yet God then went on to make David a great person – it was okay to feel and express such despair.

> How long, O LORD? Will you forget me forever? How long will you hide your face from me? How long must I wrestle with my thoughts and every day have sorrow in my heart? How long will my enemy triumph over me? Look on me and answer, O LORD my God. Give light to my eyes, or I will sleep in death; my enemy will say, 'I have overcome him,' and my foes will rejoice when I fall. But I trust in your unfailing love; my heart rejoices in your salvation. I will sing to the LORD, for he has been good to me. (Psalm 13:1-6)

Today is the pits. Things seem so pointless. The threat of this pleurodesis is confirmed when I reference Google again and find that lifespans are very limited, especially in malignant pleural effusion like mine. Sounds like such a last ditch effort to save patients. Yet I feel so well except for some small symptoms such as breathlessness after coming upstairs.

Call from a cardiovascular nurse at Auckland Hospital. I put a lot of questions to her which she didn't really want to answer. One comment gave me a glimmer of hope: 'A pleurodesis is sometimes done on air pilots because of spontaneous pneumothorax; successfully achieved, they can return to flying.' That certainly doesn't sound like a disability.

Gave myself a good talking to: said get over yourself and find a distraction. The perfect mood displacer: have been enjoying losing myself putting together our photo album from Michelle and Dale's wedding. What a wonderful visual reminder of such a special day.

> Your body is a temple of the Holy Spirit... (1 Corinthians 6:19)

Julie ~ Last night I spent a couple of hours in praise and worship claiming your healing in line with the two Orewa ladies. Felt it good to cash in on the open heaven they created yesterday and add my AMEN to it.

Today got Psalm 42 which I have adapted for you: '...Oh my God, my soul is cast down within me. Therefore I will remember you from the land of (New Zealand)... deep calls to deep in the roar of your waterfalls. All your waves and billows have swept over me... The Lord will command His loving kindness in the daytime, and in the night His song shall be with me – a prayer to the God of my LIFE... I will say to God my Rock, Why have you forgotten me? Why do I go about mourning because of the oppression of (cancer)? My bones suffer mortal agony as my foes taunt me, saying to me all day long 'Where is your God?' Why are you so cast down oh my soul? Why so disturbed within me? Put your hope in God for I will yet praise Him, my Saviour and my God.'

Sunday 9 September 2012

Julie – There is a song based on Psalm 13 that was such a comfort to me three years ago. I too expressed my despair at that time before the Lord – God appreciates our honesty before Him. But the end says,

> But I trust in your unfailing love
> Yes my heart will rejoice
> Still I sing of your unfailing love
> You have been good, You will be good to me…
> ('Psalm 13, How Long O Lord' by Brian Doerksen)

We need, then, to look up and see Him looking lovingly down upon us, longing to take us in His arms and bring us comfort and healing. The song ends with what you have claimed since the very first moment: God's goodness. Hold onto this one fact and you are entirely SAFE.

Shirley – It's really just a day-by-day thing and receiving such positive reinforcement from God's Word sent by thoughtful friends gives me something to focus on and look forward to. My head knows the truth of God's goodness but possibly my heart doesn't know it enough.

Graeme and I prayed again this evening, covering ourselves, our family and our home with the blood of Jesus. We cursed Satan and his demons. We claimed the healing and wholeness that comes through Jesus.

Monday 10 September 2012

Julie ~ I wanted to let you know that we have set specific prayer times during the coming weeks as our intercession with God specifically for you. Our faith is strong and we are so confident in our God who definitely singled you out for a purpose, and we know that He is by no means finished with the work that He has started. We want to come alongside you during this difficult time and be a support to help lift your arms when they get tired and weary.

Shirley ~ It seems that I have been depending more on the prayers and input from others rather than continually claiming God's Word and promises for myself. God wants me. God wants to directly work in my body and my mind (changing my thought-life to alleviate doubts and fears). I've spent time this morning with Him confessing and proclaiming His truths from the Word. God has so much more for me to learn and claim as His truth.

I feel totally inadequate and unprepared for any of this – and I am so confused. But I see myself as an empty vessel just waiting to be filled and there is no doubt in my mind that when He is good and ready He will fill it and direct me how to use it. I don't know much, but this I do know: true joy is found in God's presence.

> You have made known to me the path of life; you will fill me with joy in your presence, with eternal pleasures at your right hand. (Psalm 16:11)

> Praise the LORD, O my soul; all my inmost being, praise his

holy name… who forgives all your sins, and heals all your diseases, who redeems your life from the pit and crowns you with love and compassion… (Psalm 103:1-4)

Peter remembered and said to Jesus, 'Rabbi, look! The fig tree You cursed has withered!' 'Have faith in God,' Jesus answered. 'I tell you the truth, if anyone says to this mountain, "Go throw yourself into the sea," and does not doubt in his heart but believes that what he says will happen, it will be done for him. Therefore I tell you, whatever you ask for in prayer, believe that you have received it, and it will be yours. And when you stand praying, if you hold anything against anyone, forgive him, so that if your Father in heaven may forgive you your sins.' (Mark 11:21-24)

I tell you the truth, if you have faith and do not doubt, not only can you do what was done to the fig tree, but also you can say to this mountain, 'Go, throw yourself into the sea,' and it will be done. If you believe, you will receive whatever you ask for in prayer. (Matthew 21:21-22)

But he was pierced for our transgressions, he was crushed for our iniquities; the punishment that brought us peace was upon him, and by his wounds we are healed. (Isaiah 53:5)

Tuesday 11 September 2012

Graeme ~ There were private moments of total despair. Sometimes I felt as if my heart would burst with sorrow and my chest felt so restricted it was difficult to breath. But Michelle, Richard and I attempted to keep the worst of our fears and heartbreak to ourselves and not make our suffering a further burden for Shirley to carry.

Recent setbacks and the necessity of the pleurodesis procedure had been the catalyst for taking a fresh look at the whole area of praying for healing – to examine what our expectations were and weigh them against God's wishes; to consider the fact that there are many types of healing, and both small and large miracles, and Shirley had most certainly already experienced many blessings along the way. We were also experiencing that amazing peace which God gives when we ask Him for it and commit everything to Him – no matter whether the roller coaster is up or down.

Shirley and I reached a tacit agreement that we would place our future in God's hands and, as much as humanly possible, continue our life as if the elephant which resided in our lounge was not rearing up, bellowing, and threatening to crush us under its weight. It was Shirley's wish that we carry on a normal life and we endeavoured to do so trusting that she knew her limitations.

In an email to our loyal band of supporters I wrote:

It's tough, it has been very tough, but we trust God totally for the outcome – in all these things He knows best. That He is honoured in everything is our top desire. So many verses of God's Word point to healing. Please believe with us.

Yesterday's oncology appointment was an appalling experience. In essence it was a discussion about planned palliative (ugh!) treatment. The general plan is that treatment after surgery won't be rushed – with a balance considered between quality of life and controlling/slowing/shrinking the cancer cells with chemotherapy if it becomes uncomfortable.

Thursday 13 September 2012

> Heal me, O LORD, and I will be healed; save me and I shall be saved, for you are the one I praise. (Jeremiah 17:14)

Shirley – Friends came to pray with me today – they later emailed:

> Grains of sand (like the scattered cancer specks) are not able to withstand waves washing over them – they go where they're carried – and God wants His waves to wash over you. We feel you've been robbed of joy (joy of the Lord, joy in your heart). God wants to FILL you with His joy. And then, there's the verse: 'A cheerful heart is good medicine, but a crushed spirit dries up the bones.' (Proverbs 17:22) Where your joy/happiness has been robbed, stolen, taken, it's time to reclaim it. Fill your house with His praises which oppose a spirit of heaviness. Loads of love and declaring LIFE and ABUNDANCE OF JOY over you.

Friday 14 September 2012

Shirley – Dale and Michelle gave Graeme and me vouchers for Explore NZ – a half day trip out on a large catamaran searching for dolphins and whales in Auckland's Hauraki Gulf. What a wonderful afternoon – a burst of beautiful weather, heaps of dolphins and one very friendly whale that stayed with the boat for 20 minutes or so.

This evening I attended an intercessory prayer seminar (plus all of tomorrow). Words of knowledge were given to me:

You have the key in your hand. All you have to do is turn the lock. As you unlock that door you will enter into new things God has planned for you. It is the key to the kingdom of heaven, a beautiful place of peace and prosperity. Let's go there together, the King is there. You are going to meet the King on earth. Come into His presence, fellowship with Him. As you minister you are getting filled up – worship, praise, dance – this is the key. Keep doing this, you will lead others – like Esther went into the king's presence with boldness. You have desired these things. Come, enter in freshness, intimacy. You have Esther's heart – break into boldness. You will share this with others. God is here now. (Saw flight of stairs.) Step into what I have for you.

Saturday 15 September 2012

Shirley – I'm still on a natural high from yesterday's beautiful vision. Throughout my life I have always attempted to share God's message and be (however inadequately) an example of living in Christ; but I am mindful always that I am merely a vessel and pray that He works through me and guides my words. So yes, of course I would be proud to walk in Esther's footsteps.

The intercessory prayer seminar today was excellent – very informative and an interesting experience. I'm really grateful to have been able to come and share in the day and have that new awareness of the power that God gives us through prayer.

The early afternoon quiet time with prompting from the front was really helpful – I was able to touch base about a few things, submit to Him again, and a couple of new enlightening ideas came to me. But when the time came for the giving of prophecies, for some inexplicable reason, after the lady spoke over me

I felt disheartened. I felt so sad I just wanted to bawl. I stayed for as long as I could then had to leave. In hindsight I realise a strong terminal/death spirit had come over me. On the way home I gave in and just cried and felt that there was no hope of survival. I even ranted at God telling Him that if He wasn't going to heal me to stop torturing me and take me now.

It was another downer – and looking back I realised that Satan hadn't liked that some more of his strongholds were removed from my life earlier in the afternoon. So together with Graeme I confessed the words I had spoken in the car and told Satan to get out in Jesus' name. We asked to be covered by the blood of Jesus and cut off any power from the spirit of death. Immediately the dark cloud and heaviness lifted. In fact, since then I have found myself really laughing about little things – a sort of bubbling up from the gut and a new joy and release in my spirit.

Monday 17 September 2012

Julie – Yesterday morning our reading was from John. My husband read verse four and said, 'This is for Shirley: "This sickness will not end in death. No, it is for God's glory so that God's Son may be glorified though it."' (John 11:4) Hallelujah!

Shirley – This verse is coming my way from various people:

Be strong and very courageous... (Joshua 1:7)

It takes courage to stand up in the face of sickness and declare you are healed by the stripes of Jesus. There are going to be days when you'd rather hide than take another faith stand against Satan. But you can't. Because the battle of faith isn't fought once and then forgotten. If you want to keep living in victory, you have to fight it again and again.

If you're going to fight the good fight of faith to the finish, you'll have to continually draw courage from the Word of God. Get into that Word and let it change you from a coward to an overcomer. (Be Courageous, *Faith to Faith*, Kenneth and Gloria Copeland)

May the Lord answer you when you are in distress; may the name of the God of Jacob protect you. (Psalm 20:1)

Wednesday 19 September 2012

And my God will meet all your needs according to his glorious riches in Christ Jesus. (Philippians 4:19)

Shirley ~ Need to spend more time with the Lord. Need to work on such areas as disappointment and rejection.

Trust in the LORD with all your heart and lean not on your own understanding; in all your ways acknowledge him, and he will make your paths straight. (Proverbs 3:5-6)

Do not be anxious about anything, but in everything, by prayer and petition, with thanksgiving, present your requests to God. And the peace of God, which transcends all understanding, will guard your hearts and minds in Christ Jesus. (Philippians 4:6-7)

CHAPTER 7

A New Diagnosis

Sunday 23 September 2012

Shirley ~ Graeme and I have been away at Pakiri Beach, north of Auckland, for a few nights. We stayed at this amazingly creative 'arty-farty' beach house up a long, gated driveway. The house had no locks on the doors. It was a good relaxing getaway disturbed by only a few interesting creaks in the night.

We were reminded of the story of Abraham when he submitted in obedience to God because he loved and trusted Him completely. It wasn't until the last moment when he was about to sacrifice Isaac that God told Abraham not to do anything to him...

Now I know that you fear God... (Genesis 22:12)

I will surely bless you... (Genesis 22:17)

Julie ~ Trust you are having a beautiful day. Just want to tell you I took communion for each of you four today and got a real anointing for your healing.

I really feel something critical happened today. I saw you

wearing a heavy coat that just fell off your shoulders freeing you completely.

Monday 24 September 2012

Shirley ~ Today is Michelle's birthday. Twenty-two years ago, when God placed this precious soul into my care, I could never have imagined being happier or feeling more blessed. But when I look at this beautiful loving young woman today, I am in awe and thank God for giving me such an amazing daughter. I am so very, very grateful for her.

> May the God of hope fill you with all joy and peace as you trust in him, so that you may overflow with hope by the power of the Holy Spirit. (Romans 15:13)

Tuesday 25 September 2012

Shirley ~ In Auckland Hospital for pleurodesis operation. Good opportunities to talk with lovely Filipina and Indian nurses about the Lord. Also a big haze of pain and morphine.

Graeme ~ I was drained, exhausted and struggling to overcome the frustration of being forced to stand by as yet again Shirley was placed in a life or death situation that was totally out of my control. All I could continue to do was give thanks that we had our remarkable relationship with God and that I could call on His emotional support to help us get through these devastating times. We were also immensely grateful for the outpouring of love and support that came unstintingly from Shirley's army of prayer supporters, who I knew would be standing by waiting for news. So despite the undeniable fact that I was struggling to keep my own spirits up, I got to work and sent out an email:

> Just to let all you wonderful caring and praying people know that Shirley finally had her pleurodesis operation late this afternoon.
>
> With their usual professional detachment, the staff I spoke to reassured me that the operation went well, which I guess means no complications. We give thanks for the prayers raised up to our Lord.

Sunday 30 September 2012

Shirley – Yesterday I got by on just Panadol. The evening was a different story: before going to bed I took a dose of morphine but woke up at 3 a.m. in pain. Took more morphine but needed more again at 8 a.m. It's a sharp, debilitating pain that restricts breathing. I have been warned, so hopefully what I am experiencing is normal.

Michelle and Dale came up yesterday – she did my shopping and then made up a couple of meals for us, while Dale vacuumed. Bless her, she still found the energy to treat me to a manicure (prettily painted fingernails and toenails) – she's spoiling me. Graeme and I are so bowled over with the continuing miracle that we are witnessing in her. Oh that her relationship with God will be strengthening as well. Daughters are amazing and precious, but oh so mysterious – I now have some understanding of how my parents must have felt about me as I was growing up.

Healing? Having been isolated in a clinical atmosphere for several days, I felt the pressures of Satan in the air. When I got to the ward I prayed against the spirit of death which obviously has a lot of success in a hospital ward and seems to hover over the beds. In no uncertain terms I told every demonic being where to go in Jesus' name.

I'm having fun coordinating a balance between keeping mobilised to facilitate lung drainage and succumbing to the effects of morphine. And a woozy mind is not the best for investigative thought, but so much inspirational intercession keeps leading me back to the Lord to spend time with Him. God is good; I need to repeat again that He is in control and is healing my body, despite not seeing the evidence at this point in time. I long to hear the words that tell me I have received a miracle. Come Lord, quickly please, and work in me; use me as a living example to encourage the many believers, and prove your power to the sceptical ones.

Monday 1 October 2012

Shirley - I have a very noisy lung, some difficulty breathing and a lot of coughing. This all apparently goes with the post-pleurodesis territory. Being home is good because it is easier to be more mobile, which greatly aids my respiratory symptoms. I also need to keep on top of the pain as it will take four to six weeks for the artificially created pleural irritation to settle down and fix the two pleural layers around the lung together. The collapsed lung is also re-inflating again after another 800 millilitres of fluid was drained away.

I visited my GP today and had stitches removed, so all is looking good at present.

That sounded like it was all about me unfortunately. Really it's all about God and the fact that He is the most amazing Heavenly

Father. He is the One for our focus, and He's the One who listens and hears and answers our prayers. No obstacle is too large for Him – and so we trust Him.

This beaut verse was shared earlier this week by my old flatmate and nursing colleague and remained with me long after I had read it. I was left with the sense that I don't have to struggle or fight or even use up all my energy because the Lord will carry me:

> I have made you and I will carry you; I will sustain you and I will rescue you. (Isaiah 46:4)

Tuesday 2 October 2012

Shirley – Had a bit of a setback today. I'm under instruction not to do any heavy lifting and have been, up till now, a good girl. Yesterday, however, I carried two not unduly heavy photo albums from bedroom to dining room so I could start making up a photo board for Richard's twenty-first birthday party. Halfway there, the books morphed into a ton weight and I had this sudden sharp pain in my diaphragm – it felt like a tear. I took my fullest dose of morphine, lay out on the La-Z-Boy chair and phoned the specialist. Have to keep up the pain relief, so it's hard to say if the pain's improving or what. So annoying. Resting, resting, no photo albums, be good. Hope I haven't undone anything. Don't want to mess up what they're trying to achieve with this pleurodesis procedure.

Wednesday 3 October 2012

Shirley – Sometimes I feel that I have nothing left to give – no more resources to call on to carry me through. In all honesty I feel like throwing my hands up and giving in; then I think about it and recognise it as an action of despair that is an indication of surrendering to God. Whenever I ponder and then create a space, either God's words speak to me or I am directed to a passage in a book (same thing?). So the following came as no surprise today:

> 'To you I call, O LORD my Rock; do not turn a deaf ear to me. For if you remain silent, I will be like those who have gone down to the pit. Hear my cry for mercy as I call to you for help, as I lift up my hands toward your Most Holy Place.' (Psalm 28:1-2)

David turns to God in his time of trouble, but it's important to note how he turned to God: David turned to God in surrender. Lifting up hands is a sign of surrender. It is an acknowledgement that you are before someone more powerful. Lifting up hands is also a sign that you have gotten to the end of yourself; you have nothing left to give. In fact, in a negative sense, it can be a sign of giving up. In the positive sense, it is a sign of surrender as we give up to God. Surrender to God is always a healthy place to be. David also turned to God with respect: 'O LORD my Rock… your Most Holy Place'.

What is our language to God and about God like in difficult times? I pray that we continually acknowledge God's goodness, His faithfulness and His sovereignty in every season. I pray that we acknowledge this to ourselves and to others. (Steve McCracken)

'I am still confident of this: I will see the goodness of the LORD in the land of the living. Wait for the LORD; be strong and take heart and wait for the Lord.' (Psalm 27:13-14)

Don't give up! Your final chapter has not yet been revealed – it has been written – but it has not yet been revealed. God is ordering your steps if you are submitted to Him. God is for you, He is not against you. God delights in you and is always working for your best. (Steve McCracken)

Friday 5 October 2012

Shirley – Today we heard the devastating news that Graeme has bowel cancer. I can't believe I am writing this – it seems so unreal. This just feels like too much to bear. I am shattered. God has known about this all the time. We certainly don't understand His ways – but His ways are (somehow) perfect. We are stunned. Speechless!

> My grace is sufficient for you, for my power is made perfect in weakness... (2 Corinthians 12:9)

> Trust in the LORD with all your heart and lean not on your own understanding; in all your ways acknowledge him and he will make your paths straight. (Proverbs 3:5-6)

Sunday 7 October 2012

Shirley – Today we shared Graeme's news with Michelle, Dale and Richard. My precious children – they'd already been dealing with a roller coaster of emotions – so many reassurances followed by disappointments, constantly living with a juxtaposition of fear and hope; the stress must have at times seemed intolerable. But they were, after all, our children and Michelle reacted with her generous loving heart on her sleeve, crying, 'It's so unfair.' Richard immediately switched over to dealing with the practicalities of the situation and putting our minds at rest. They are both remarkable and have a core of strength that has never been more evident than now. Knowing that God will sustain them is the one true thing that keeps me from utter despair.

It's so hard – so very hard – yet in other ways okay because we know that God is in control, even though humanly speaking this is all totally beyond us.

> 'Sing to the Lord, you saints of his; praise his holy name. For his anger lasts only a moment, but his favour lasts a lifetime; weeping may remain for a night, but rejoicing comes in the morning… You turned my wailing into dancing; you removed my sackcloth and clothed me with joy, that my heart may sing to you and not be silent. O Lord my God, I will give you thanks forever.' (Psalm 30:4-5, 11-12)
>
> Praise in a season of weeping is unnatural naturally but is always natural spiritually. There's something supernatural about praise; it changes environments. There is something faith-filled about praise, and faith always pleases God.
>
> Your current season is not your final season. God delights in turning things around, but He does so in His timing. God's timing is always the best timing. Difficult seasons are not wasted seasons – God is always working for our good. I pray your praise releases the season of God that you anticipate. (Steve McCracken)

Monday 8 October 2012

Shirley – I woke feeling that God is stripping everything away from me, my sense of who I am has shifted on so many levels: no urgency to be somewhere I am needed, such as Bible in Schools; my self-esteem – all my previous lovely straight hair looks like a mop and my body is a crisscross of scars; my poor prognosis – despite my unyielding belief; and now Graeme. It's more than I can bear, Lord. And what about our children? But when I shared my feelings with Graeme he calmly replied, 'God can do a new thing. It's okay.' Wow. I recognised my negative thoughts as lies of Satan.

Graeme – It was certainly not that I was attempting to be glib about the new development in our situation, but it seemed unimportant when weighed against the broader implications. My immediate concern was not about having cancer myself but the impact of this additional trauma on Richard and Michelle. What if I died? The enormity of such a situation would be unbearable for them. And what if they were to lose both of us?

Naturally I was concerned for Shirley too, but I knew she had a wide circle of friends and would have good support if anything happened to me. At this point I felt that what she most needed from me was quiet reassurance and to just get on with it. I was like a duck on a pond: calm and unruffled on the surface and paddling like crazy beneath it.

Just for the record, this was the sequence of events around my cancer diagnosis:

The North Shore Hospital Board had a free bowel screening programme for 50 to 74-year-olds, and I thought I should take the opportunity to get myself a clean bill of health. This led to a colonoscopy where it was discovered that I had a 'moderate size cancer' which could cause an obstruction within six months if left untreated. As you can imagine, our initial reaction was shock and disbelief at the double whammy. We realised that our reaction over time could potentially be very negative or we could choose to turn to our loving Heavenly Father. By and large, we responded with the latter and totally trusted Him in all this and believed His Word. We then made a conscious point of surrounding ourselves with positive people – none of this death and dying stuff.

> O Lord my God, I called to you for help and you healed me. (Psalm 30:2)

Tuesday 9 October 2012

Shirley – In the midst of all this we find time to rejoice. This I find hard to believe: my little boy is officially all grown up – today is Richard's twenty-first birthday. We get to formally celebrate the sharing of 21 fantastic years with our precious caring son. And to give thanks for the strength and maturity that is demonstrated in everything he does. What could make a mum more proud?! Thank you, Lord.

> 'My soul will boast in the Lord; let the afflicted hear and rejoice.' (Psalm 34:2)
>
> There is something powerful about the testimony of a praising Christian in the midst of difficulty. We want to celebrate what God has done in us. We want a testimony.
>
> For some it's time to stop waiting for the opportunity to

have a testimony on the other side of your difficulty and understand that your greatest testimony can be now. Praise in pain honours God very much and it releases a fragrance of God that is attractive to others. Your testimony can be greater in trouble than in a time of peace. That which you think hinders the work of God just might be the best environment for God to get the most glory through you, especially if your attitude and speech reflects a deep confidence in the God you love. So today, put on the garment of praise, let it come out of your lips so others can hear and be amazed at the testimony you have right now. (Steve McCracken)

Julie ~

May the God of hope fill you with all joy and peace as you trust in him, so that you may overflow with hope by the power of the Holy Spirit. (Romans 15:13)

Graeme has been your strength and staunchest supporter throughout these arduous years, fighting your battle with you; to have him join you in the fray (so to speak) is just too much. No words can express our feelings right now for you both.

Yes, the signs show the enemy's footprints everywhere. Speechless! Yes, we are speechless. All I can say is that you must have been doing something good and valuable for the kingdom to have attracted such evil intention. Fight we must and FIGHT WE WILL!

It's devastating news and certainly you guys are under attack. It's understandable the way you are feeling. We will certainly be praying strongly and conducting warfare on behalf of you both. I know His purpose is at work within you, as He's guiding your life with wisdom and love. There are greater things than you can imagine ahead of you and there's a great God walking beside you.

It's hard (and knowing you I am sure you are already doing it) but I encourage you to fill your house and your heart with praise. Keep at it. Praise is also warfare – the enemy hates to be around it. When you really don't feel like it – when you feel like you can't – you just make that decision and do it. God totally comes through and raises your strength, hope and faith, and gives you peace. As your spirit exalts His Name and declares His goodness, He lifts you from where you feel that you're lying – sometimes face down in the dirt. He brushes you off, He mends your armour, and as you turn your whole focus to Him, the enemy is defeated.

I don't want to sound glib, but what the enemy seeks to destroy – the chaos he brings – pales in comparison to what God can do; and we know that God causes all things to work together for good for those who love Him – those who are called according to His purpose (Romans 8:28). That's you guys.

Wednesday 10 October 2012

Shirley ~ This evening Graeme and I went to a meeting at a Christian centre. The preacher was only available to see us briefly, but it was time well spent and we have a further private appointment with him next week.

Thursday 11 October 2012

Shirley ~ I woke up this morning and my throat felt empty – released from the dryness and irritation that was causing the constant need to cough. All the ulceration and swelling since the intubation had completely gone. Praise the Lord. Not sure yet about any other changes.

> 'I sought the Lord, and he answered me; he delivered me from all my fears.' (Psalm 34:4)
>
> God always answers us when we call. Sometimes we don't hear much but that is not evidence that God is not listening and answering. My lack is not evidence of God's lack. God is always faithful to who He is and He is a God who always listens and who always answers. Sometimes His answers are different to what we want to hear. Sometimes His answers come from different places than we expect. But I am convinced that He always answers. David's insight here is that God delivered him from all his fears – not all his problems.
>
> Many times our fears are greater than our problems. The truth is that God never gives us a spirit of fear. In fact, Perfect Love – God Himself – drives out all fear. I believe one of our greatest victories in life is to walk without fear in times of difficulty. This is very honouring of God and powerful against the enemy. (Steve McCracken)

Julie – I want to encourage you again to praise in the midst of pain and anger and doubt. Our God is the same yesterday, today and forever, and He loves you all as much now as He did when He died on the cross for you. Your prayers and our prayers are being heard, and I'm praying for you and Graeme and your children for peace that surpasses all understanding and a sense of God's almighty power and sovereignty in the midst of what is happening in your lives. May you be encouraged and take refuge in the Lord – your Rock, your Fortress and your Deliverer. May He lift you up and raise you high; may He give you deliverance and triumphs; and may you know His mercy and steadfast love.

Graeme – All our friends, and the extended army of people who were praying for Shirley, knew how staunch her love for Jesus was. They all knew that her life was a testament to God, and in everything she said and did, she asked for His guidance and influence. Her faith was unquestionable. So when others reminded her to send up praise even though she was at her lowest point, she did not take this as a reflection on her behaviour or inference that she was not already doing so. Instead, she welcomed every comment and embraced every offer of support, appreciating and understanding their sincere intent.

Saturday 13 October 2012

Shirley – It was Richard's twenty-first birthday party this evening and what a great party it was. It would be difficult to say who had the best time – he and his friends, or the adults who were there to show their love and support.

All our close friends and family know how much I have enjoyed preparing special food and baking for family events, and understood that I would be feeling frustrated and redundant that I couldn't cope on my own. The overwhelming result was a small army of people offering their help in various ways. They were amazing and we were all delighted with the results this joint effort produced. Blessed yet again!

Before the party, we were visited by a couple who shared their own story about battling cancer. Six years ago the husband was healed from metastatic lung cancer. He gave us some valuable advice, and of course his own testimony was an enormous encouragement. We are blessed with wonderful friends and a God who has an extravagant love for us.

> Those who look to him are radiant; their faces are never covered with shame. (Psalm 34:5)

> Consider it pure joy, my brothers, whenever you face trials of many kinds, because you know that the testing of your faith develops perseverance. Perseverance must finish its work so that you may be mature and complete, not lacking anything. If any of you lacks wisdom, he should ask God who gives generously to all without finding fault, and it will be given to him. (James 1:2-5)

Julie ~ I have been pondering what you said about feeling stripped of everything (8 October) and feel the Lord wants you to know that while you still have HIM then you are not stripped of everything. While all your activities gave you a sense of usefulness and fulfilment, He is saying all you need at this time in your life is Him. Let your circumstances drive you deeper into Him and He will meet all your needs. In His eyes you do not need to be *doing* to be loved and accepted by Him. Just rest in Him, my friend, and He will be all in all to you.

Monday 15 October 2012

Shirley ~ Wondering if I am being pruned by God. I feel as if I have been poked and prodded, cut and sliced, stitched and patched and I'm a perfect advertisement for the walking wounded. All worth it, of course, if God has a greater purpose for me.

No one sews a patch of unshrunk cloth on an old garment, for the patch will pull away from the garment, making the tear worse. Neither do men pour new wine into old wineskins. If they do, the skins will burst, the wine will run out and the wineskins will be ruined. No, they pour new wine into new wineskins, and both are preserved. (Matthew 9:16-17)

Tuesday 16 October 2012

'The tongue has the power of life and death…' (Proverbs 18:21) And, 'Reckless words pierce like a sword, but the tongue of the wise brings healing.' (Proverbs 12:18)

Shirley ~ Today Graeme and I went to see the preacher who we had previously spoken to at the Christian centre, for some words of knowledge and his healing ministry. He spoke about the power of words. At this time in my life, I confess that the concept is easy – it's during the execution that I so often fall down. Controlling errant thoughts has not always been my strongest characteristic (indeed Graeme often lovingly teases me about my spontaneity and tendency to have ideas pop up at the most unlikely of times). Need to look at this and confess as God shows me.

The pastor followed this with a time of ministry, routing out demonic forces and bringing in God's healing and wholeness to our bodies. Saying the cancer has no right in our bodies – that 'we are the temple of the living God…' (2 Corinthians 6:16)

Julie ~ Remember the song It Is Well With My Soul that was written by Horatio Spafford, who lost his four daughters on a ship crossing over to Europe. I believe some of the words to the song are, 'When peace like a river, attendeth my way, when sorrows like sea billows roll; whatever my lot, thou hast taught me to say, "It is well, it is well, with my soul."'

I know that God would like you both to know that even though we continue to pray and believe for your healing, more important than that is the health of your soul. And it is well with your soul. From the day we are born, we are dying. We give so much attention to our bodies, yet some give no thought to their souls. So we continue to pray for your bodies, but it is your soul that is of greater worth to God. And it is well with your soul. Completely well!

Thursday 18 October 2012

Shirley – Graeme is going for an MRI Scan at 4.30 p.m. Once again I cannot believe that I am able to announce such frightening words with such conviction that it is a formality only. And even if there is still a manifestation of the cancer, 'by his wounds we are healed.' (Isaiah 53:5) Hallelujah!

Julie – It is really important to be in an atmosphere of people who believe with you. Our focus is God's word. Jesus said, 'It is finished...' (John 19:30) Our salvation and healing is complete in Him.

> 'Are not two sparrows sold for a penny? Yet not one of them will fall to the ground apart from the will of your Father. And even the very hairs of your head are all numbered. So don't be afraid; you are worth more than many sparrows.' (Matthew 10:29-31)
>
> I reject the lie in your life that says you are worthless. I

speak against the lie that says nobody cares. I silence the lie that says your situation is hopeless and nothing good will happen. I rebuke the father of lies who incessantly attacks and speaks contrary to the truth.

You were born of God's will and intention. You are wonderfully made. You have a hope and a future. You have value and significance. You are known by God and loved by God. God Almighty is for you and nothing can stand against you and prosper. God Almighty has given you authority over all the enemy's powers. God Almighty has started a good work in us and He personally is committed to its completion.

So stand up, shake off the dust of intimidation and the lies of the deceiver and start believing the truth of what God Almighty has declared about you. You are more than a conqueror through Christ. You are a child of the Most High God. You are a friend of the King of Kings and the Lord of Lords. You are seated with Christ in heavenly places. You are called, forgiven, accepted, valued, loved, empowered and filled with the fullness of the Eternal One True God. (Steve McCracken)

Friday 19 October 2012

Shirley ~ Today I went back to the Southern Cross Hospital to have the port-a-cath (for chemotherapy) reinserted in my right jugular vein (just like old times). Fairly uneventful, except it has left me feeling light-headed and a bit dizzy. Probably just need a good sleep.

As the surgeon's appointment isn't until October 29, and we couldn't hold our breath that long for the results of Graeme's MRI and CT Scan, we recruited the help of our GP. Oh blessed

Lord, the results say that NO METASTASES are seen in his bones, body organs or lymph nodes. Naturally we find this very encouraging and an enormous relief. A consistent description was 'unremarkable'. A confined 2.5 cm thickening was seen in the bowel wall. A clearance report would have been the one to be really excited about but we trust God totally for His timing and healing.

Someone recently reminded me of a popular quote: 'When the going gets tough, the tough get going.' I can certainly relate to that, particularly if I put it into my own terms and exchange the second 'tough' with 'God'. In the same vein, I've often heard that people show their true colours when their backs are against the wall – well that's true as well. We feel as if we have been stripped bare and every little blemish or imperfection has been exposed. We are certainly learning a lot about ourselves.

It has also been an interesting exercise for us to pour over God's Word as the truth in conjunction with medical truth. Against all odds, it has been a really fruitful time for us, providing a unique opportunity to build up our faith and focus on our Lord.

Biding time waiting for further appointments is frustrating and unsettling, we feel as if we have been frozen in a time-warp. So we have decided on a short break; we are leaving tomorrow morning and heading south for a week. We plan to stay with close friends on their peaceful rural sheep farm (no other sounds but the rustling of breeze through the many trees; no cars, no blaring TVs, no sirens piercing the still night air, and no other unwanted intrusions – oh bliss). Graeme hopes to get into the great outdoors.

Saturday 20 October 2012

Shirley – At 2 a.m., needing to go to the loo, I got out of bed and promptly fell back onto it. The slight dizzy unstable feeling I had after yesterday's surgery was now major and I staggered from one handhold to another looking like a marionette without its strings. I made it to the bathroom only to find that the toilet seat had magically turned into a see-saw. I negotiated my way back to bed and sprawled over Graeme, waking him to announce that I couldn't walk properly. Short story is that he called an ambulance and I was taken to North Shore Hospital where they investigated for a stroke (a possible complication from port-a-cath insertion can be a blood clot which then lodges in the brain) or a possible brain tumour – which we were relieved to know showed as negative on the brain CT scan. Oh what a night.

CHAPTER 8

Wonderful Respite

Sunday 21 – Sunday 28 October 2012

Shirley – We finally got away to Raetihi, where Graeme managed to add an enjoyable day skiing at Turoa, as well as some other scheduled activities. I spent my time meandering around the farm being amused by the antics of dozens of frolicking lambs and catching up on some reading. It was great to spend time with my friend and enjoy her generous hospitality. At the end of four days I was so relaxed I felt boneless. Graeme, on the other hand, was totally invigorated and felt as if all his muscles were humming.

A significant part of this jaunt was being on the byways and keeping off the highways. We travelled back via the 15 km Forgotten World Highway from Taumaranui to Stratford then had a night at Waitomo. As we travelled we played worship CDs which ministered into our hearts.

There's so much going on, so much spiritual warfare to be done. We are claiming healing – Jesus won the VICTORY on the cross and Satan was defeated. Each day we are proclaiming God's Word aloud, particularly scriptures about healing.

There were two spiritual growth areas for me during this week.

When I was prayed for and anointed with oil, the word 'fear' was suggested. At the time I couldn't relate, but during this week God has been showing me some areas of fear in my life and I have renounced them.

> For God did not give us a spirit of timidity, but a spirit of power, of love and of self-discipline. (2 Timothy 1:7)

God is good. This has given me a new sense of release and confidence in God's strength.

The other has been forgiving myself – a rather new concept for me. One particular area God showed me is where I have allowed myself to be victimised by somebody outside our family who intimidates me and has constantly put me down. Strange as this may sound, since working through this issue I have gained an incredible sense of liberation and the person no longer has the power to hurt me. It was a process as simple as this: acknowledging the damage inflicted on me, forgiving the perpetrator, and letting it all go as I gave it over to God. It was a major leap forward in personal empowerment.

I came home determined not to start chemotherapy yet, despite having a port-a-cath inserted. I am not ready to face it and hate to contemplate the fact that my quality of life will be reduced by the potential side effects of peripheral neuropathy. When in doubt: I have asked God to show me what I should do. Not sure how He will do that.

Sunday was our wedding anniversary and we spent time reminiscing and quietly enjoying being in the shelter and warmth of each other's company. We are so very blessed.

Monday 29 October 2012

Shirley – Graeme and I each had an appointment. First, we went to North Shore Hospital for an appointment with the bowel surgeon. Lots of helpful detail, probably information overload for Graeme. But we feel reassured to have a Christian surgeon. He is also Director of the Bowel Screening Programme where Graeme was diagnosed with cancer. We understand he is very experienced in this specialty area, and certainly our discussion with him convinced us we are being offered good options and explanations.

Second, we were told by my breast surgeon, who inserted the port-a-cath, that she took a further breast biopsy during the surgery. The results showed adenocarcinoma to the dermal lymph layer on my left breast – despite having undergone 25 doses of targeted radiotherapy nearly two years ago and being told that the chances of cancer reappearing in that breast were almost non-existent. Her conclusion: 'You need to start chemotherapy immediately.' So God has answered a prayer I prayed yesterday. Just not the answer I wanted to hear.

I feel scared, scarred, stitched and patched. I have been pricked, prodded and cut. And I feel weak when I should feel strong. And fear when I should feel faith. At the moment I am feeling very fragile and very human and in need of God's reassurance. And of course he heard me and attempted to lift me up and lighten my load with humour. The book I was reading flipped open to this:

> When a bookstore owner told me a woman had stomped into his shop, angry, slamming one of my books on the counter, I knew exactly what he was talking about. I wrote that Jesus

may have had pimples. He may have had bony knees. But I said, 'One thing's for sure, he was, while completely divine, completely human.'

There's something safe about a God who never had calluses. There's something majestic about a God who never scraped his elbow. But there's also something cold about a God who cannot relate to what you and I feel. Rejection? He felt it. Temptation? He knew it. Loneliness? He experienced it. Death? He tasted it. And stress? He could write a best-selling book about it. Why did he do it? One reason. So that when you hurt, you'll go to him and let him heal you! (Max Lucado, *In the Eye of the Storm*)

For we do not have a high priest who is unable to sympathise with our weaknesses, but we have one who has been tempted in every way, just as we are – yet was without sin. (Hebrews 4:15)

Tuesday 30 – Wednesday 31 October 2012

Shirley – For the next two days Graeme and I both felt 'blah' (no other word for it really). Takes a lot to get either of us down but this was a lot. We are so disappointed about my latest cancer development; we were at a loss for words and bewildered by the seemingly conflicting messages God was sending me. But by the end of this time we recognised Satan's hand trying to defeat us, so we quickly resumed our spiritual fight.

Starting tomorrow I will be having 18 weekly doses of Vinorelbine with Herceptin added three-weekly. Bad news!

And for the good news! Pleurodesis chest x-rays show that the procedure has been very successful, the pleura has fixed well together and my lung has inflated back to normal size and position. Shortness of breath is now history. Graeme's main memory of the appointment is that it is now safe for me to fly – so watch this space.

As you keep praying, we keep believing and trusting our awesome God.

Monday 5 November 2012

Shirley – Had my first dose of chemotherapy (Herceptin and Vinorelbine) today. Before previous chemotherapy I was loaded with heavy anti-emetics and steroids, but not this time, supporting the information given that this is a less severe chemotherapy treatment. During the infusion I had sharp pains in the middle of my back, and heaviness and pain all around my upper body. I very much appreciated the intravenous Dexamethazone (steroids) administered to relieve the pain.

Our take on this situation is that Satan doesn't want me healed. He stabbed me right in the middle of the lumbar-thoracic where all those sclerotic spots were seen on x-ray – a last ditch attempt to discourage us. But that's exactly where God is healing me. We certainly need to keep up our warfare prayer.

Julie – 'No weapon forged against you will prevail…' (Isaiah 54:17) God has already won the victory. God alone gets the glory.

Wednesday 7 November 2012

> There is a time for everything … a time to weep and a time to laugh… (Ecclesiastes 3:1,4)

Peace in the Storm

Shirley ~ Friends visited this morning to share a message they had received. They reminded us about Paul's shipwreck where God protected him from the viper (Acts 28:3-6). They believed God showed them this in relation to me and as a picture that my body also will be protected from chemotherapy damage. After they left I realised that the intense itchiness on the soles of my feet and palms of my hands that I've had since chemo was gone. Thank you, Lord.

Email arrived from Michelle:

> I've been thinking about how a lot of things come down to our perception of them. So instead of being upset about what we can't change we should think about what opportunities all these challenges are giving us.

That is so true. And wow how perceptive and mature my daughter has become.

Friday 9 November 2012

> to bestow on them a crown of beauty instead of ashes, the oil of gladness instead of mourning, and a garment of praise instead of a spirit of despair. They will be called oaks of righteousness, a planting of the LORD for the display of his splendour. (Isaiah 61:3)

> Praise be to the name of God for ever and ever; wisdom and power are his. He changes times and seasons; he sets up kings and deposes them. He gives wisdom to the wise and knowledge to the discerning. He reveals deep and hidden things;

he knows what lies in darkness, and light dwells with him. (Daniel 2:20-22)

Graeme ~ Faced with Shirley's trials, my own illness seemed insignificant, but the added stress for both of us was incapacitating. We knew we were not in a good space and needed help from someone older and wiser, so we transferred all our problems over to God and resolved once and for all to trust that He would take care of us and sort it all out. Much of this particular period is thankfully a blur, so I again refer back to an email I sent responding to the many caring enquiries regarding my medical development:

> With no obvious symptoms or warning, my diagnosis of a small to medium colorectal tumour was very much a big surprise (of the not-so-good variety).
>
> After discussion with the surgeon at North Shore Hospital, I am booked for an operation on Wednesday 28 November. It has been decided that no chemotherapy is required to shrink the tumour (huge relief – very selfish, but after watching helplessly while Shirley suffered through her treatments, I feel very blessed to be reprieved from a similar experience). Any further treatment will depend on the histology results from the operation, so we are again in limbo doing our least favourite thing – waiting.
>
> I have been reading an inspiring book called *10 Hours to Live* by Brian Wills. He was a professional tennis player and at only 22 years was struck with Grade 4 Lymphoma. A tumour in his abdomen grew overnight from golf ball size to nine-month pregnancy. He was given 10 hours to live. His family's journey was about immersing themselves in prayer,

God's Word and praise and worship CDs. Excellent principles, I highly recommend this read.

Apparently I will most likely lose weight (been physically active so not a lot to spare), and I'll be really wasted for four to six weeks. Chances are I could become a skeleton covered with skin. Anyway, such is life and we go with the flow.

Tuesday 13 November 2012

'God is our refuge and strength, an ever-present help in trouble.' (Psalm 46:1)

Our fear can distort our perceptions and make us see the answer as just another problem. God's best always requires facing what we fear. The disciples were in a boat lashed by waves. Jesus called Peter to come to Him on the water. But there's always a moment after you step out in faith when you hear, 'What if I'm not up to this?' Peter heard it, and the waves began to engulf him. Panicked he called and Jesus immediately rescued him. Peter wasn't drowning, he was learning and growing. When you walk by faith, even your failures will lead to success. So step out with Jesus; He won't let you drown. (*Word for Today*)

Shirley ~ If God says that my number of days is up then I accept that. But when I contemplate that eventuality, my heart aches at the thought of leaving my family and the huge weight of grief it would place on them. My life has been so rich and full and I want to live it out to the fullest extent, being constantly excited at the thought of what God has in store around the corner. Obviously I cannot make such a monumental choice – I must continue to give it over to God and patiently wait for His decision. This is undeniably an interesting season in my life but one where God seems to be saying, 'Okay girl, I want all your attention.' Well, He sure knows how to get it.

Friday 16 November 2012

Shirley ~ I feel an excitement which must be like that experienced by a new Christian saved by grace. When I think of all Jesus achieved on the cross I'm overwhelmed with gratefulness to Him and filled with love. I feel like singing and I intend to keep fuelling this wonderful feeling with positive language and uplifting reading material. When you feel this good you want to shout it to the rafters and bore everyone you know talking about it.

Our regular prayer time with friends this morning was very rewarding – we had a great time covering lots of areas but specifically praying for healing. Everyone was in great form (must be contagious) and the fact that I was so 'perky' was commented on.

Sunday 18 November 2012

Shirley ~ Over the weekend I noticed that the gland in my neck, which was measured four by four centimetres across by the oncologist, has shrunk enormously. Also the newish dermal eruption of adenocarcinoma on my left breast has reduced visibly. All praise and glory to God. Very exciting.

Some friends from overseas stayed with us overnight and contributed their faith and energy to some very special prayer times. We focused specifically on praising and honouring God and building up our faith, believing in the healing that God has for us. Praise God that from this date I no longer had pain or stabbing in my back.

By his wounds we are healed (Isaiah 53:5)

Wednesday 21 November 2012

Shirley – Just a quick note to keep you updated on the chemotherapy front and how we are. It doesn't come naturally reeling off lists of aches and pains when I'd much rather talk about the remarkable work that committed Bible teachers in public schools are achieving, for example. But here we are and we sincerely do appreciate all your prayers. We know that with God all things are possible and so much other amazing truth that is set out in His Word. We love faith-filled prayers that draw you to God, and when we benefit from the spin-off from those prayers we are truly blessed.

Monday this week was the third chemotherapy session (15 to go) and already my white blood cell count is below the normal range. So exposure to coughs, colds and other bugs needs to be kept minimal. The immediate obvious side effects of the current drugs are very little compared to the toxicity of my chemotherapy exposure two years ago. However, I did have an unpleasant reaction the first week, so subsequently am being given a steroid infusion before the chemotherapy infusion. The first day is, therefore, not my brightest day. A sleeping pill taken that night seemed to be the best way to ensure some sleep and afford a semblance of normality for the rest of the week. Otherwise life continues as usual.

I was privileged yesterday to assess a CRE Bible teacher for accreditation. What a joy when a child told the Bible teacher, 'I really like Bible. It's better than great.' What joy when school staff members are supportive to the planting of seeds of God's Word alongside our Values Programme.

Thursday 22 November 2012

Shirley – On several occasions lately I have shared with others about an enormous decrease in the size of the gland on the left base of my neck, the size of adenocarcinoma of left breast, and minimal back discomfort since focused prayer. All I receive is an almost disbelieving stare and scepticism. No excitement or encouragement. It's as if they don't want to give me false hope so they do nothing. It's very discouraging, almost patronising. Well does God have some surprises coming up for them!

> 'Then they understood that he was not telling them to guard against the yeast used in bread, but against the teaching of the Pharisees and Sadducees.' (Matthew 16:12)
>
> Jesus told His disciples to be careful who they listened to. I think He would say the same to us in the Church today. People's words are influential. Just because someone is a Christian does not mean it is beneficial for us to listen to their teaching. We need to be wise. If someone contradicts what the written Word of God says, don't listen to them. If someone is characterised by negativity, don't listen to them. If someone is focused on judgement, don't listen to them. If someone is sceptical, don't listen to them. If someone pulls others down, don't listen to them. If someone is more politically correct than biblically correct, don't listen to them.
>
> If someone is talking about God in a way that whets your appetite to know Him better, listen to them. If someone stirs your faith to believe for the supernatural, listen to them. If someone stirs your heart with compassion to love others more, listen to them. If someone stirs you out of complacency,

listen to them. It's time for us to listen to the God-honouring voices. (Steve McCracken)

Monday 26 November 2012

Shirley – This is a big challenging week. (Reading that back to myself I thought, 'that's a bit of an understatement,' but it is almost beyond me to describe what we are going through.) Graeme's surgery is coming up on Wednesday and it's my fourth chemotherapy today. But on the positive side, we now have a beautifully decorated Christmas tree to enjoy. It's a family tradition to put it up a month before Christmas and Michelle and Dale came and did the honours for us. It was a joyful occasion filled with old 'remember when…?' stories that sent us into fits of laughter.

I seldom let my circumstances get on top of me but today I was caught unawares. I was suddenly overwhelmed with the enormity of the situation. Here I was with the IV infusion needle in my port-a-cath and a small mobile trolley by my bed with a syringe of 'poison' (Vinorelbin) that kills off tissue if you get it on your skin, with my stomach churning worrying about Graeme's upcoming operation. Picture me lying there, a magazine hiding my face, attempting to suppress huge gulping sobs. Tears were streaming down my face and running into the neck of my blouse, and of course (when you most need them) there were no tissues in sight. Not a picture for the family photo album, but who cares – having a good cry when needed is meant to be healthy.

Had my three-weekly appointment with my oncologist today. I asked for his comment on my 12 November high tumour marker blood test result. He said that his best indicator at present was the shrunken above-collar-bone gland mass and the virtually disappeared adenocarcinoma on my left breast. He suggested that the tumour marker was raised because there was a high incidence of dead cancer cells in my blood stream. Oh really! Praise the Lord.

Graeme ~ After so many years together, Shirley and I were pretty good at non-verbal communication and I know for a fact that at this point we were both so concerned about adding stress to each other that we suppressed our fears as much as possible. It was a balancing act between admitting vulnerability and talking ourselves up. The mind plays tricks on us and we often have difficulty recalling past details that are unpleasant so I am grateful to Shirley for recording all the missives we sent out to our growing band of supporters. This is an excerpt from an email I wrote during that period:

> I have stopped work and am slowing down for a couple of days prior to my operation. I'm told I'll be in hospital for a minimum of five days and likely longer while I learn to use and cope with an ileostomy bag (yuck), but hopefully it will only be for the predicted three months. The purpose of this barbaric procedure is to give my bowel a rest while it heals. If I insisted, I could go without the bag but there's a 10 percent chance the new 'plumbing' would leak and cause an infection in the abdominal region, which would turn into a major and be very hard to cure. I know of someone who ended up like that and he had over five months off work, whereas the usual is about six weeks. To reverse this will mean another operation and another month off work, presumably in three months' time.

About then Shirley should be finished her current chemotherapy cycle – who knows, we might even grab a short holiday somewhere. Fortunately my time off runs into the Christmas holiday period so I'll actually end up with seven weeks off work by the time I plan to go back on January 14. A test run for retirement perhaps?

Interestingly enough I do remember that I was pretty relaxed about the actual operation, just struggling a bit with the post-operative process. One requirement was a drastic change in diet during the healing stage and I was put on a strict soft food regime, to which I responded, 'Oh goodie.' But fortunately for me, ice cream was on the approved and recommended food list.

Looking back, I have no doubt whatsoever that it was our faith and trust in the Lord, combined with the friendship and involvement of so many wonderful people expressing their interest and concern, which made the journey easier to bear. So although (of course) we had our moments, we didn't feel depressed or sad. Rather it helped us to become more concerned and interested in other people who also had health issues. Undeniably, the word 'cancer' does strike fear into our heart (studies suggest that it is often the word itself that kills people, rather than the actual symptoms), but it is just one of many diseases that can strike us and they all cause disruption to our lives.

I know that I am a more compassionate and caring man today than I was at the start of this journey.

CHAPTER 9

Appreciating Each Other

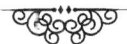

Wednesday 28 November 2012

Shirley – Graeme's bowel resection surgery is today. He is amazing – so calm and matter-of-fact about the whole thing. What an example – it makes me feel like a snivelling, whining, feeble malingerer by comparison.

We are so surrounded by prayers it is overwhelming and I never doubted for one moment that he would do well, that God is with us totally and in control. But, oh boy, I found waiting while he was in theatre exceptionally tough, despite the many calls and texts of support. However, we were in capable and experienced hands and, sure enough, immediately after the three-hour operation, Graeme's surgeon phoned to say that he was pleased with the outcome.

So the end result was worth waiting for, and when I was able to visit Graeme later in the evening, I was immensely encouraged – he looked amazingly good and it was so wonderful to see him.

Before the operation, Graeme was so impressed by the groundbreaking research and development which is being achieved in this area of cancer that he volunteered to take part in a trial that looks at the amount of keyhole surgery used for bowel resections.

So typical of him to be thinking of how he could benefit others through his own experiences.

Thursday 29 November 2012

Shirley ~ By the next day, Graeme was already making noises about coming home. Such a quick recovery, we suspect, has something to do with his physical fitness but I (more than anyone) am aware that the impact of major surgery will doubtless hit him over the next few days. So I am prescribing lots of rest.

We are now back into our all too familiar pattern of waiting for histology results from the surgery. Once the location of tumours and lymph nodes and associated tissue are analysed (hopefully next week), the surgeon can be more definite about the outcome. He said that the tumour was quite small, only one and a half centimetres, quite different to the three-centimetre mass photographed and measured during Graeme's colonoscopy over a month ago. It will be an interesting point to discuss but we have no doubt that with God nothing is impossible.

In the short term, Graeme will be adjusting to life managing an ileostomy, which he isn't relishing. However, he has already met with a great support network in the hospital and there are specialist nurses available for home visits in our Rodney area. Before going in for surgery he was saying that he hoped to be able to talk to other patients who are struggling with their own situations – ever the opportunist and optimist we so admire.

Wednesday 28 November – Tuesday 4 December 2012

Shirley ~ Graeme's time at North Shore Hospital was uneventful

– he was positive and looked and felt pretty darn good as well. I had difficulty sleeping all week and was so grateful that Michelle, Dale and Richard were able to fill in and visit as much as they could. Finally Graeme came home and it was such a relief to have him here. We so much wanted to be there for each other but neither of us was in a position to do much about it – so we cracked feeble jokes about being the walking wounded and ended up laughing. But as my brother wrote by email: 'Look after each other. No one else can do it as well.'

Thursday 6 December 2012

Graeme ~ Shirley and I had always been close friends, enjoying a deep and meaningful intimacy and open communication – we liked one another and supported each other in everything we did. We needed no reminder of our wedding vows promising to stand by each other 'in sickness and in health' – it was the core of our relationship – but we often joked that the balance had shifted somewhat at this juncture.

It was never an issue with me: sick or well, happy or sad, good or bad, I loved Shirley just the way she was, and my only regret was that I couldn't fix this for her. I have always been blessed with the ability to compartmentalise my mind and place my attention where I choose, and this, I am sure, enabled me to cope at a time when so much was going on. I simply placed my affairs in God's hands and focused on being there for Shirley.

I recovered from my own operation quickly, and with dire warnings of the consequences of overdoing it ringing in my ears, I was home after only a few days in hospital. We kept thanking and praising our Lord that the tumour had been found so early, and began to prepare for the next stage, which involved a six-month period of chemotherapy treatment to zap any remaining cancerous cells.

For me it was a wake-up call to stop and smell the roses more often and to be more sensitive to the needs of others rather than getting caught up in the doing and busyness of life.

Friday 7 December 2012

Shirley ~ We have both had a few emotional moments as we struggle to come to terms with our present position. It feels so unfair. It seems as if every time we overcome one hurdle another higher one is thrust in our path. The latest for me has been weakness and immobility in areas where there is massive scar tissue. For the last few days I have been struggling with left arm lymphoedema. Thankfully a visit to a specialised massage therapist gave me some relief and got me back on track.

Usually I am the one going to bat for the underdog and fighting for some good cause. It is a very uncomfortable feeling for me to be the one considered in need of help, and it has taken a huge paradigm shift in attitude – it is far easier to be the one doing the giving than to learn to sit back and do the taking. It's not that I don't appreciate every little bit of kindness and the many thoughtful ways people have found to show their support, but it is not an easy adjustment.

Of course I never expected it to all be roses, but sometimes life can be so unfair. Earlier this evening, feeling overwhelmed and totally over it all, for the first time (in complete desperation) I vented my frustration on God. I pleaded and begged Him for answers. Where have I failed you? What do I have to do? Have I not had enough faith and hope to please you? Have I misinterpreted your word and gone against your wishes? Because, God, something is seriously out of whack here: although (and for this I give heartfelt thanks) there have been many small miracles along the way, clearly I am not healed.

Oh well, dummy spit over. God will understand, and I figure He can handle my outburst and understand my disillusionment at being perceived and treated by many (including those in the medical profession) as being in a slow, irrevocable, downward decline. I hate it.

Shortly afterwards I read *Word for Today* and felt a renewed focus:

'Let the Word of Christ dwell in you richly…' (Colossians 3:16)

Press in. Draw into a more intimate relationship with your Heavenly Father. If you don't, you won't make it. If you do, you will see more glorious outpourings of God than you can imagine. Those who don't do what the Spirit says will go from disaster to disaster. But those who do will defeat the disasters and turn them into glory, in Jesus' name.

The first step in drawing closer to God is to realize that you know God first in His Word. Time spent meditating in His Word is time spent with Jesus. Letting the Word dominate our thinking is to allow the Holy Spirit to have control over your mind. As you do that your feelings will fall into line.

Saturday 15 December 2012

Because you have so little faith. I tell you the truth, if you have faith as small as a mustard seed, you can say to this mountain, 'Move from here to there' and it will move. Nothing will be impossible for you. (Matthew 17:20)

Julie ~ 'Thou art coming to a King, large petitions with thee bring, for His grace and power are such none can ever ask too much.' (John Newton)

Shirley ~ I am attempting to fill my heart and mind with nothing but praise and flood my soul with God's love. I will overcome. I will be gracious in defeat if that is what is required of me.

Tuesday 25 December 2012

Shirley ~ Christmas day. Such a perfect day, it sets the scene for us all to celebrate and remember the birth of Christ. Our family unanimously voted to hold Christmas at our place so we could honour all our old traditions and hopefully create some new memories. It ended up with 18 people for lunch. Everyone pitched in and, with very little contribution from me, pulled it all together and produced a fabulous banquet.

Graeme ~ Christmas Day 2012 – 23 years of celebrating the birth of Christ with my amazing wife. As she sparkled and shone with happiness at being surrounded by so many people she treasured and who loved her, I realised that this could be our last Christmas together. I watched her intense focus whenever someone was talking to her and her animated responses; I saw her eyes dance every time they landed on her adored children and marvelled at the closeness between each of them; I ached for her that she had been unable to make her usual contribution to the menu; I saw how beautiful she still was even though her body had been through so much invasive surgery and her luxurious hair was a thing of the past; I watched and I wondered at the gift I had received to have enjoyed this woman's companionship and love for so many years. I didn't want to contemplate the thought of losing her.

Monday 14 January 2013

Shirley – Chemotherapy Dose 12 today (six to go). How I'd love to stop having this poison. Unless I'm not seeing the signs or listening carefully enough, God has not told me to stop so I'll keep going to the eighteenth dose unless He intervenes. This is definitely a case of living by faith not by sight as we don't know exactly what my physical condition is in terms of cancer. I'm guilty of sometimes being so focused on the current problem I forget to see the glass half full and give thanks that there have already been so many miracles along the way: the four by four centimetre supraclavicular gland gone; the left breast adenoma gone; the back-stabbing pain gone. But lest I forget, whenever I share testimony of God's healing and goodness I get a niggle in my back as if Satan is saying, 'How do you know you are healed?' I fight back and mock him, 'By Jesus' wounds I am healed,' and tell him to get out in Jesus' name.

In the midst of all this, someone will always ask the million dollar question: 'If you believe that God is healing you, why did you continue with all this harsh treatment?' The truth is that no one will ever know what the overall outcome would have been medically if we had made different choices. At each step along the way we believed that if we prayed for guidance before, during and after every decision we made, then we were proceeding in the right direction.

I also remind these people that miracles come in all shapes and sizes and often occur without fanfare, and that healing can happen on many different levels. But the expectation is of course that it should be all or nothing. Well, I for one am very happy with the lesser offerings and totally accept that complete healing may not be mine on this plane.

And so back to my current status with regard to the latest dose of chemo: Even though I sleep well each night (with the aid of tablets) I'm so whacked that I'm pretty much wasted most days. In between essential ongoing tasks (which are good for me) and finding time for a short walk, I spend a lot of time horizontal. My excuse is a combination of weak muscles and a rather foggy brain. Ironically, so many people are saying that I look great (my loyal husband agrees) after seeing me at social events or church. We've worked out that I have a surge of adrenaline for the duration of these occasions and then crash into a big heap when we hit the car or arrive home.

Fortunately there is always another side to this story. You see the little 'c' (cancer) has a formidable competitor in the big 'C' (Christ). God is on our side and He knows what He is doing and we just trust Him totally. But we also believe that He is even more interested in us having a growing relationship with Him than for us to be physically healed. There are so many words in Scripture that encourage us to trust God's absolute goodness and love, despite the many tough things going on around us all. And we never overlook the fact that God is not the author of those tough things.

Monday 21 January 2013

> In his heart a man plans his course, but the LORD determines his steps. (Proverbs 16:9)

Shirley ~ Got back from chemotherapy today and did the usual horizontal crash. Was so over it just getting up our stairs! Anyway I started shivering and shaking, so I bundled up with cardigan and blankets and hoped I would come right. But things deteriorated and I was feeling worse by the minute. Eventually I clicked that I could have a fever so took my temperature: 38°C (which is when you have to report). With vivid memory recall of my last ghastly reporting experience two years ago, I reluctantly made the call.

I was told to take two Panadol tablets. So I put on socks and another layer of warm clothes and went back to bed. Next temp was 38.6°C and I was convinced I was doomed for another hospital visit. They asked if we had any antibiotics in the house. Who does that? Then I suddenly remembered I'd bought two sets of antibiotics for our proposed Europe trip. And remarkably they were the right ones. What a relief, I got to stay in my own bed where I could actually get some sleep without being stabbed with needles (my veins apparently aren't the most obliging). It was basically another write-off Monday, which I was starting to be mentally prepared for each week.

Graeme ~ It was almost two months since my operation and I'd just had my first clinical check-up. Seemed all was good and they were happy with my recovery (not half as much as I was of course). I must admit that I was surprised at how tired I was and having to resort to afternoon nana naps was totally out of character. It took me a full month to feel more or less right again, but in the scheme of things that wasn't too much of a price to pay. Here's a description I wrote at the time:

> The next stage was chemotherapy, which I took in tablet

form. I got my first batch of tablets at the end of January and then had eight cycles of three weeks (six months), taking tablets for the first two weeks followed by one week off, before repeating the cycle. It's very much an unknown how I'll react to it – some people are really sick and others have almost no reaction. Either way I'm expecting to keep on working.

I was offered a choice of medicine and method of delivery: tablet form, intravenously or via a port-a-cath (like a pin cushion inserted under the skin in your upper chest with a tube direct into the jugular vein). I chose the tablet option as it should be easier.

Following that I have to wait about six weeks for an operation to reverse the stoma. That takes me through to mid-September when I'll need another two to three weeks off work. So by then the whole process will have taken almost a year.

One interesting fact to come out of the chemotherapy discussion is that it only increases my chances of surviving and being alive in five years by 7.5 percent. Seems an awful lot of pain and inconvenience to endure for a modest percentage gain.

I was offered an additional drug that could have non-reversible side effects of tingling or loss of feeling in the hands, and other skin problems. It had to be administered via port-a-cath. This chemical only increased the survival percent by one percent, so it really wasn't that difficult a decision, the risks clearly out-weighed the potential benefits.

This is my second week back at work. I must admit that after three days I felt like I had never been away. Colleagues who held the fort for me did an outstanding job and I didn't come back to any major unfinished business. With the first six months of the year a busy time for me, I'm already working at full steam to make sure I stay in control of my work schedule.

That was an overview of my journey to date. Whilst I continued to feel stronger and stronger each week, Shirley was suffering from the cumulative and ongoing build-up of her weekly chemotherapy. She needed a lot more rest and sleep with every passing week and still had six more doses to go. We could see an end in sight but it was a long, tough haul for her.

Our enduring hope was in the Lord Jesus, knowing He was not surprised by all that was happening. Through this He was drawing us closer to Himself and teaching us to rely on and trust Him with our future.

Tuesday 29 January 2013

Shirley – Graeme started chemotherapy today. My heart aches for him and I pray that his experience with this type of treatment will not be as traumatic as mine. I've always found one of the most difficult things to deal with in life is to watch someone you love being ill or experiencing hardship, and being unable to ease their pain. I would gladly have those extra treatments myself than watch my darling husband endure all this as well.

> 'We live by faith, not by sight.' (2 Corinthians 5:7) 'I do believe; help me overcome my unbelief.' (Mark 9:24)
>
> To 'walk by faith' enables you to enter the realm of supernatural possibilities, because Jesus said, 'Everything is possible to one who believes' (Mark 9:23). It isn't rooted in

self effort, but in God's unlimited power and unchanging Word. The Word of God, received and residing within you, continually produces faith within you.

The moment you act your faith springs to life, inviting God to move on your behalf. But why does God seem to hold back on breakthroughs? God is building a solid foundation under you so that you'll be able to handle the pressures that accompany His blessing. Anything that's made well is made slowly. Anything that's worth having is worth fighting for.' (*Word for Today*)

Monday 4 February 2013

Shirley ~ The accumulation of this poisonous chemotherapy is rather overwhelming and fatigue has well and truly set in. Only five weeks to go but it feels more like a lifetime. Days run into days. But, praise the Lord, it could all be a lot worse. Although the stabbing pain has gone, my back gets tired and needs strengthening. We're thinking it may be the effect of scar tissue. Who knows?

Graeme is totally amazing in how he is handling this whole thing – he just keeps on keeping on like the Energizer battery bunny. Nothing is ever allowed to put him off his stride for very long and his optimism is contagious. Thank you God for this man in my life who lifts me up and inspires me with his unwavering faith and stoicism in the face of whatever obstacle is thrown in his path, and is the most wonderful role model our children could possibly have.

Monday 11 February 2013

Shirley – With great reluctance I endured my fourteenth dose of Vinorelbine today. We have been specifically praying about cutting short the prescribed 18-week course because of increased numbness in my feet and mouth (nothing to do with putting my foot in my mouth), painful and weak knee joints, excessive fatigue, difficulty concentrating, and other more easily reversible but uncomfortable symptoms.

A friend took me over to the hospital for treatment. She told me that at 5 a.m. this morning she was woken by a persistent knocking in her bedroom ceiling. Eventually she decided that God wanted her to pray for me, so got up and did just that – then the knocking stopped. I feel so encouraged when I hear that others are called to pray – it's a real team effort and friends are being drawn to God too. What a privilege to be one of God's people.

Wednesday 13 February 2013

Shirley – Graeme and I were invited to have more prayer ministry this evening at the Christian centre we had previously attended. What a beautiful couple with such a sincere desire to see people drawn to God and healed. We always leave their company promising ourselves to return again soon, as being around this type of energy is as good as a tonic.

I need to keep being reminded of how important it is to spend time with God. I particularly love this passage about what I refer to as the Martha/Mary equation and often remind myself (when I am in my Martha persona) that I would be far better off emulating Mary.

As Jesus and his disciples were on their way, he came to a village where a woman named Martha opened her home to him. She had a sister called Mary, who sat at the Lord's feet listening to what he said. But Martha was distracted by all the preparations that had to be made. She came to him and asked, 'Lord, don't you care that my sister has left me to do the work by myself? Tell her to help me.' 'Martha, Martha,' the Lord answered, 'you are worried and upset about many things, but only one thing is needed. Mary has chosen what is better, and it will not be taken away from her.' (Luke 10:38-42)

Friday 15 February 2013

Shirley ~ A visit (and help with the gardening) from a friend – a joy to my soul, chatting and talking about what the Lord is doing in our lives. We got on to the mystery of God, the gift of His unconditional love, and the fact that His way is perfect. It is His sovereignty, it's His grace, not necessarily understandable to us, why He spares and heals some and chooses to take others home. We trust Him.

In the evening, Graeme and I called into the supermarket on our way to visit friends for dinner. While I was in the toilet (ha ha – of all places) I heard the words, 'Reclaim the land.' Well Lord, you've spoken to me in many unusual situations (this one could take the cake) and I trust this is from you (I checked there wasn't someone in the next cubicle practising a political speech). So yes, once I work out the full meaning of what you are telling me, I will attempt to 'reclaim the land'. I did wonder if it was a metaphor for getting back to a firm foundation (my feet on the ground?) or did it mean I should move on – that God is opening those doors of opportunity.

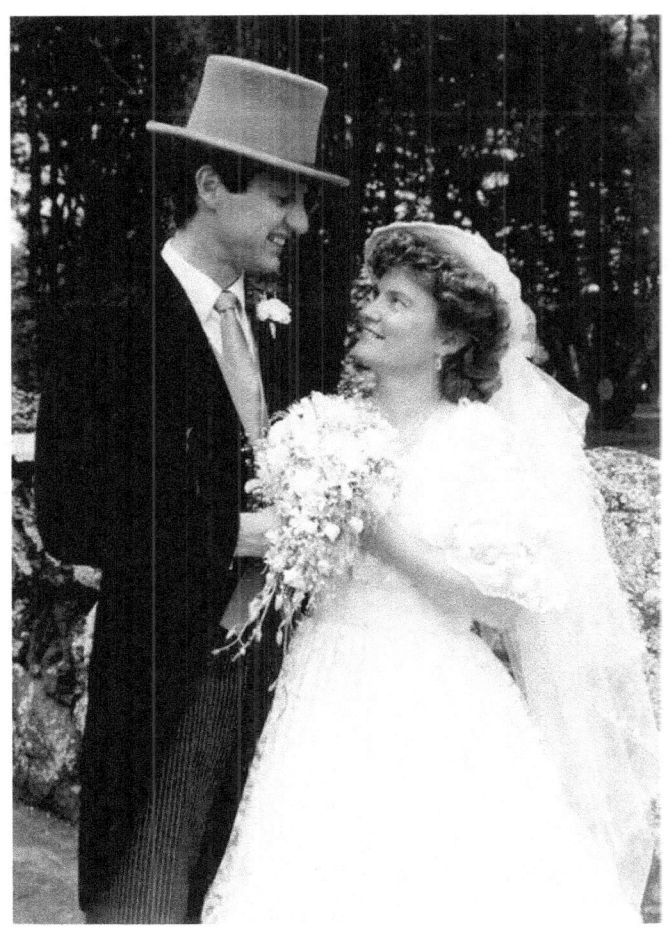

Graeme and Shirley on their wedding day, 1989

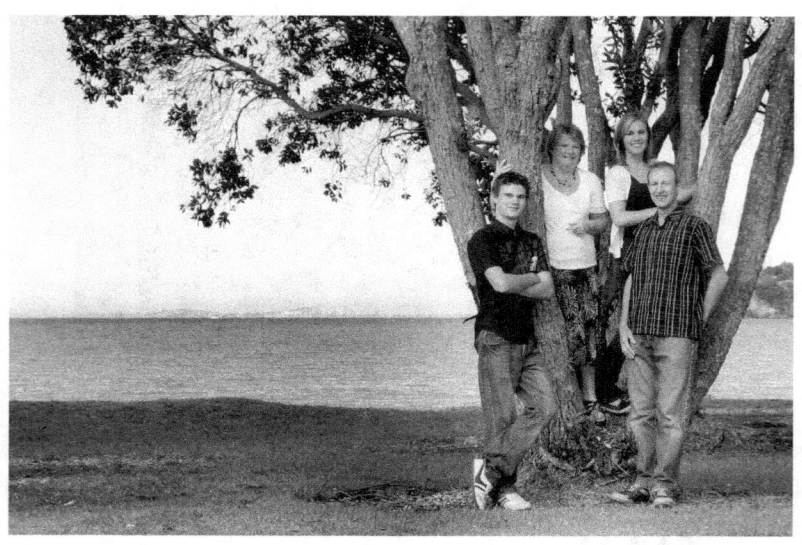

The Dando family – Richard, Shirley, Michelle and Graeme, 2008

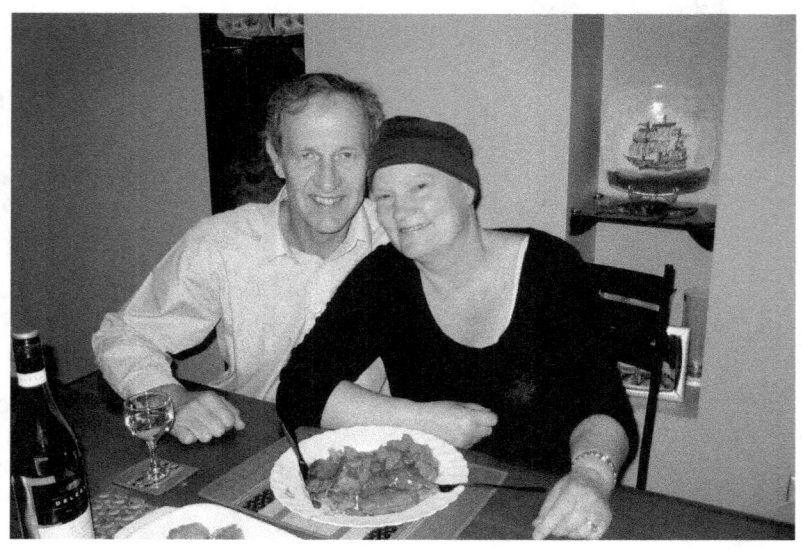

Twenty-first wedding anniversary, 2010

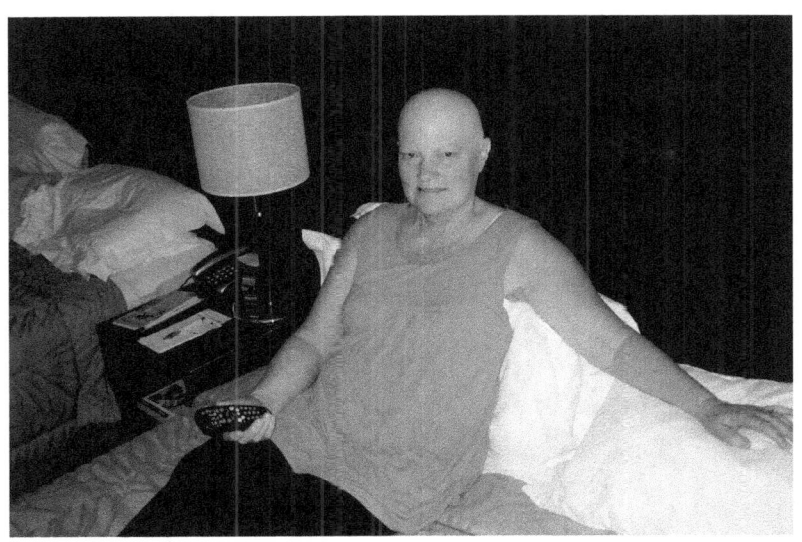

The bare head look, 2010

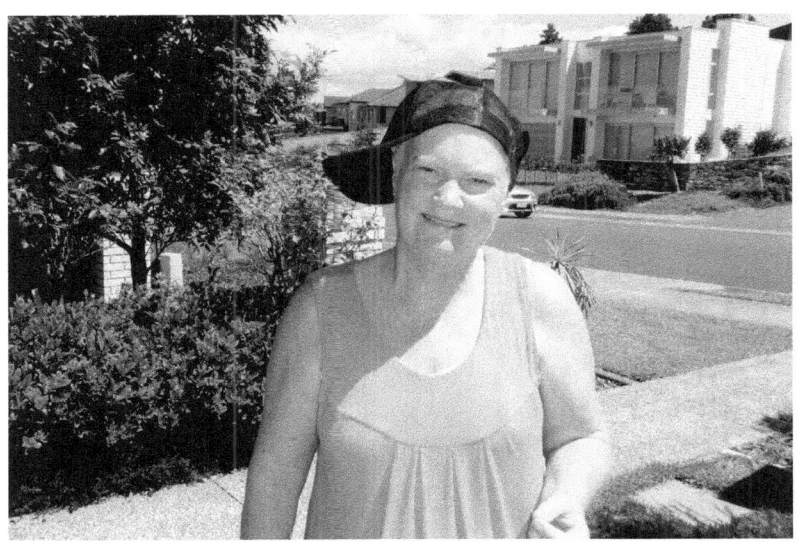

Post-chemo hairdo, 2011

Peace in the Storm

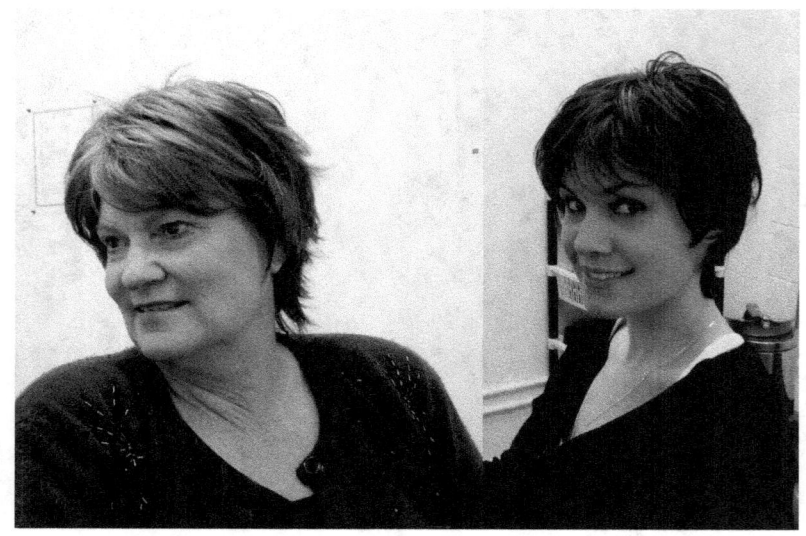

Wig shopping with Michelle, 2010

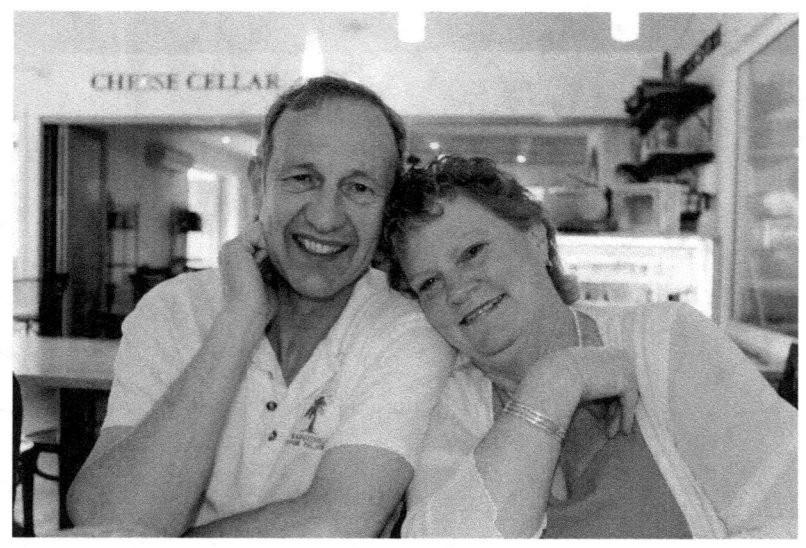

Graeme and Shirley, 2011

Photos

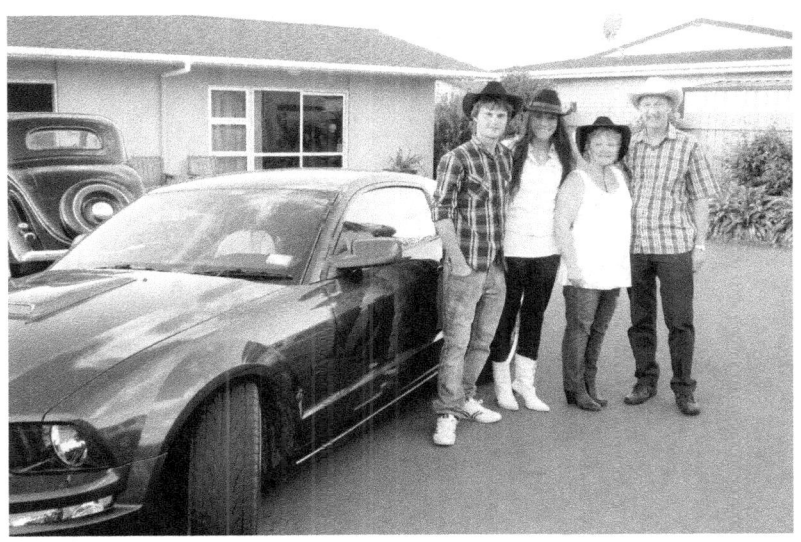

Graeme's Mustang, 2012

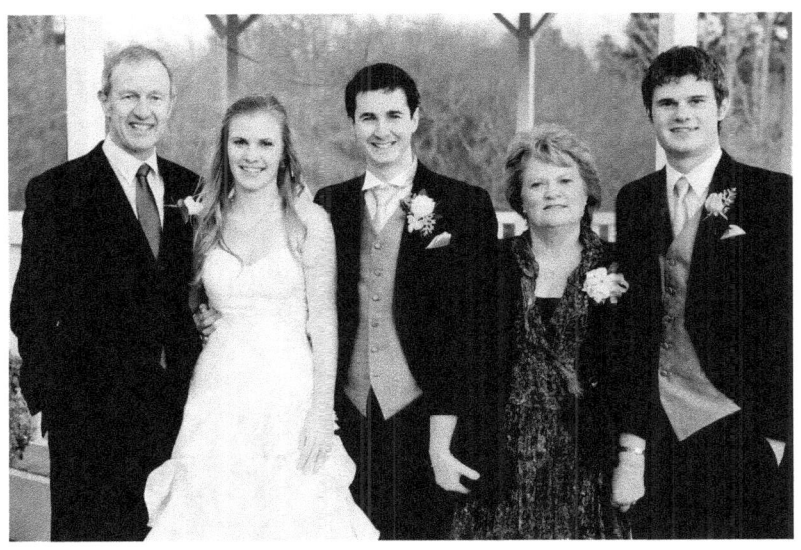

Michelle and Dale's wedding, 2012

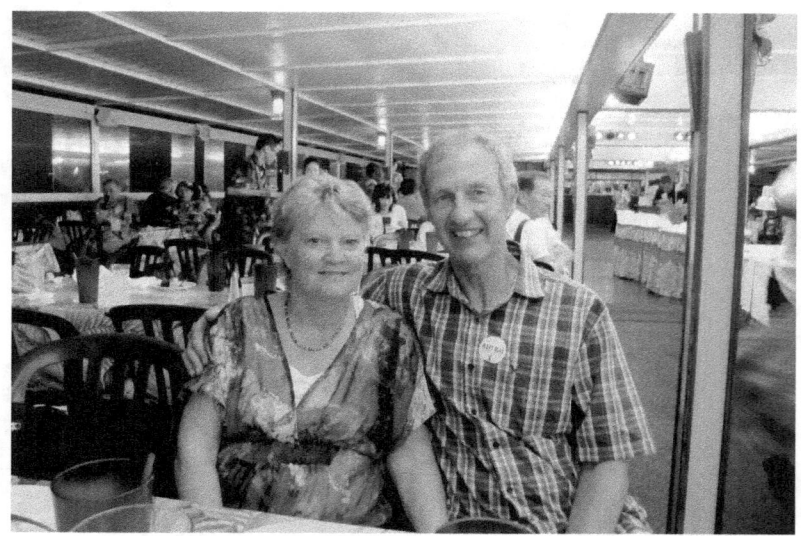

Twenty-fourth wedding anniversary in Hawaii, 2013

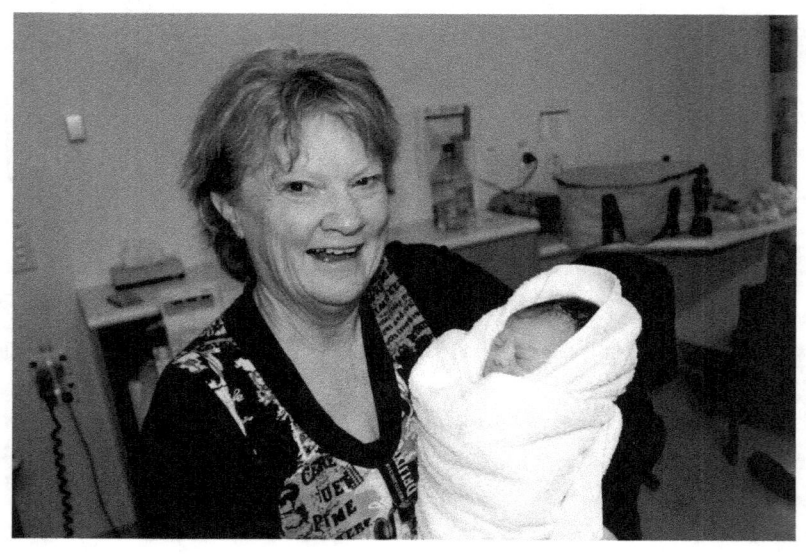

First grandchild, Jasmine, 2013

Photos

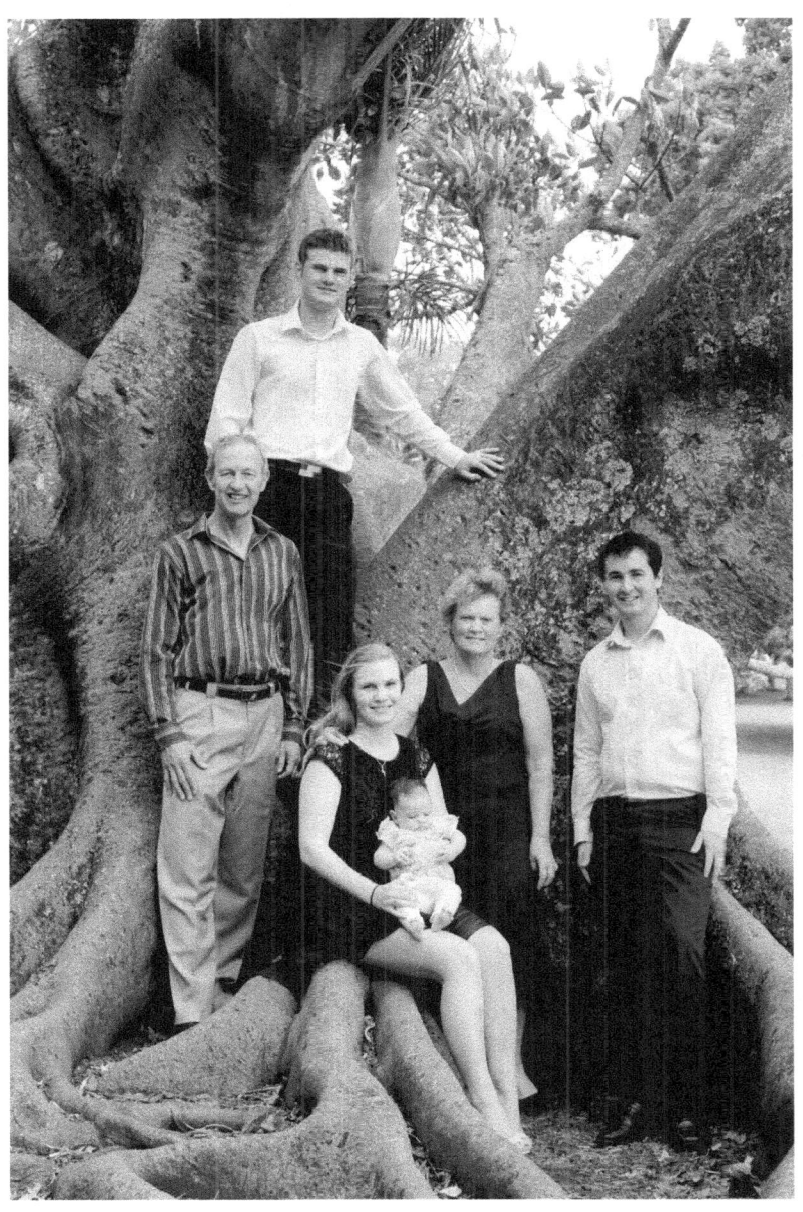

A family photo in Cornwall Park, 2013

Peace in the Storm

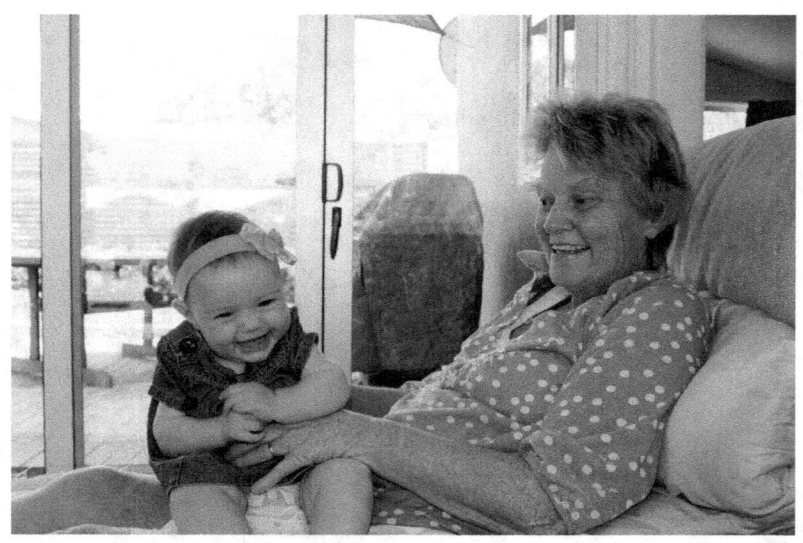

Last family holiday, Pauanui, 2014

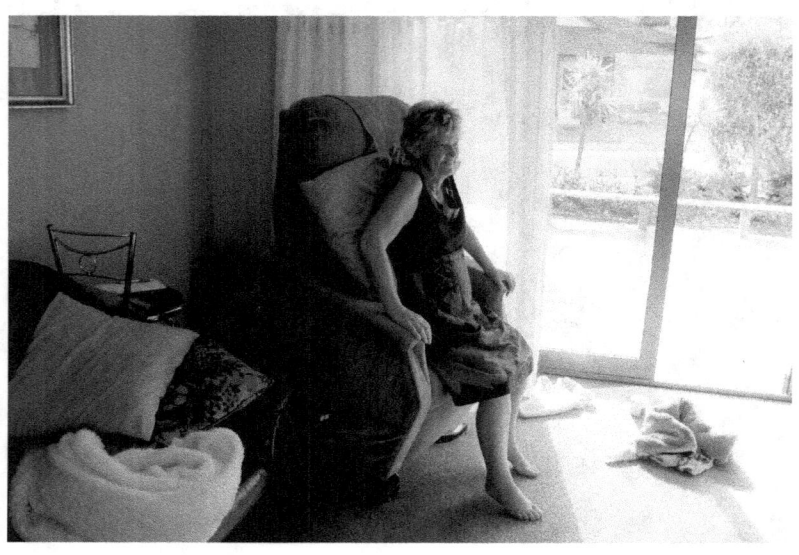

Shirley being tipped out of her electric recliner chair, 2014

CHAPTER 10

Treatment Concluded

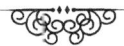

Monday 18 February 2013

Shirley – Today I stopped chemotherapy. Wait, let's have that in capitals: TODAY I STOPPED CHEMOTHERAPY. I flatly refused to have Dose 15. When Graeme and I kept our appointment with the oncologist he was at first hesitant to agree, then said that he understood our reasoning. He confirmed that my symptoms would only get worse if I continued and be more difficult to relieve. He suggested that I pick up on the three-weekly Herceptin and have it ad infinitum, but when I gave my reasons for not wanting that either, he conceded that he could see my point and once again reluctantly agreed. So yay! I'm free of chemotherapy. Hallelujah.

Herceptin reasoning:

- I had Herceptin with the six other chemicals in 2010. The reason given was that Herceptin was the 'wonder drug' that would kill off and destroy any random cancer cells that had escaped detection. Time has shown that those cancer cells weren't destroyed because they went on to metastasise in the pleura, lumbar thoracic spine and pelvis.
- Other women I know who have had Herceptin have not

survived. One was at the point of experiencing the serious side effect of heart problems. When Herceptin was stopped she died soon after from cancer.
- Another friend has had a lot of Herceptin and her cancer has continued to spread. She is now in hospice dying with multiple brain tumours.
- Extensive googling has shown that there is not a lot of confidence out there that Herceptin is really the wonder drug it is being portrayed as.
- God has told us 'You are healed' from several sources and we have an assurance in our hearts. The oncologist's previous comment that 'many people keep taking Herceptin because it makes them feel that they are doing something about the cancer' isn't how I feel. God is 'doing something about the cancer' and I have my trust in Him.

Friday 22 February 2013

Shirley – Following on from the 15 February entry – 'Reclaim the land,' I had put it to the back of my mind because I knew God would show me the meaning in His good time.

So this morning at our prayer time when this verse was mentioned – 'A nation [locusts] has invaded my land, powerful and without number…' (Joel 1:6) – I wondered if I could compare this to the aggressive cancer that invaded my body some years ago? And then there was 'I will repay you for the years the locusts have eaten…' (Joel 2:25)

I thought about God's words to Moses in claiming Canaan:

Drive out all the inhabitants of the land before you. Destroy all their carved images and … idols, and demolish all their high places. Take possession of the land and settle in it, for I have given you the land to possess. (Numbers 33:52-53)

Admittedly, still a mystery but hopefully the message is filtering into my subconscious and will process itself.

Sunday 24 February 2013

Shirley – This morning when I spoke to God I told Him that I needed reassurance about being healed. This afternoon I received a text from a friend:

> 'Beloved in the Lord. I want you to know that it is well. It is well and it is well.' That's what the Lord says. I thank my God if that was of comfort. I was sitting having a cup of tea and a thought just came through my mind that I needed to give you and Graeme that message.

The friend then followed up with a phone call and prayed a beautiful prayer of healing and restoration for all our family:

> They who wait upon the Lord will renew their strength.

Tuesday 5 March 2013

Shirley – Physiotherapy today. We are working on trying to release the toxins from my weak leg muscles and other areas. The physio worked on my back quite specifically, which I felt concerned about but decided to say to the Lord: 'Okay. Your Word says I'm healed. We have many affirmations that I'm healed. I give it to you.' As I was lying there I had a picture of Jesus, surrounded by cloud and light, with his hands out towards me saying, 'You are healed. You are healed. You are healed.' Wow. Thank you Lord, thank you Lord.

Graeme is really not well – has taken the day off work. He's very dehydrated and has no motivation (probably the most concerning aspect, as it is so not him). He's had continuous watery diarrhoea for over a week and vomited three times since the weekend. Phoned the hospital and they told him to come in for intravenous fluids and rehydration. He stayed overnight. He was annoyed that this was necessary despite determinedly drinking Fortisip, Gastrolyte, his usual water laced with lemon juice, and eating small portions of what he disparagingly calls his 'baby food'.

> May the God of hope fill you with all joy and peace as you trust in him, so that you may overflow with hope by the power of the Holy Spirit. (Romans 15:13)

Saturday 9 March 2013

Shirley – We had a lovely surprise visit today from former neighbours who arrived shortly before another couple we had been expecting. Okay. Well God knows what He's doing. I was delighted to find that the two wives got on very well and we all shared so many spontaneous God moments. Impromptu occasions such as these are often far more successful than meticulously planned ones.

God knows our needs so much. We had been given a contact number for a community dietician and followed it up later that afternoon. We were very grateful for her professional expertise on how best to deal with Graeme's current very fragile bowels (the result of chemotherapy). She was not only knowledgeable and helpful but also generous – she insisted we call her any time in the future when we needed advice. It's a great relief to know that people such as her are only a phone call away.

Sunday 10 March 2013

Shirley – Just talking to God today about my tendency at times towards a critical attitude, and as is often the case, I came home and read the following (a nudge in the right direction):

> Man's focus is so often on change, whereas God's focus is far more on relationship. People want to change leaders: politicians, civil leaders, church leaders, school leaders, employers and coaches. We see all that they do wrong. We know a better way of doing things. We understand what they are so ignorant about. In fact, if I can be completely blunt, often our desire for others to change smells more of pride than godliness.
>
> But how about God? Is He focused on the same thing? God wants us to pray for and give thanks for all those in authority because He wants us to play a part in seeing them come into relationship with Him. And this is why He wants us to live lives that are quiet and peaceable, rather than critical and antagonistic... it's all about providing the best chance of people coming towards God and not being pushed away from God by religious fanatics who carry placards and pitchforks. (Steve McCracken)

Monday 11 March 2013

Shirley – Ultrasound and check by breast surgeon this morning.

In the car on the way down to Milford this morning I continued to mull over verses I had just read:

> Are not five sparrows sold for two pennies? Yet not one of them is forgotten by God. Indeed, the very hairs of your head are all numbered. Don't be afraid; you are worth more than many sparrows. (Luke 12:6-7)

I clung to the value God puts on me/us. I clung to the truth that God is in control and I can trust Him. I wasn't afraid of the outcome of the mammogram/ultrasound because God knew it all already. Every thought led me further and further into an amazing peace.

Well, wonderful news. Earlier this week I had a regular breast ultrasound which came out with clear results. My breast surgeon came along to radiology and checked out previous obvious cancer spots: a four by four centimetre lymph node and a reasonably large skin growth (which had prompted the urgent start to chemotherapy). Ultrasound confirmed that both problem areas are clear. Her comment: 'The chemotherapy has been very effective. I guess it also reflects what is going on inside your body.' I reminded her that 'a lot of prayer has also gone into this so you can add that to the equation.' She just smiled politely – she's heard that from me before.

Tuesday 12 March 2013

Shirley – This evening Graeme noticed that his right ankle was very swollen. At the hospital on Sunday the registrar had quickly checked his calf muscle for DVT (deep vein thrombosis/blood clot) and said he was okay. Now it looked considerably worse.

I rushed to my computer and good old Google and put 'Capecitabine' (his chemotherapy drug) in the search box. There were numerous examples showing that one of the severe side-effects is potentially fatal DVT. Panicked, I leapt to the phone and called the oncology ward to talk to the doctor. They told me to bring him in. By now it was 10 p.m. and we were staggering tired so I was grateful to Richard for offering to do driving duty.

After they left, I lay in bed unable to sleep and overcome by a suffocating feeling of dread. I couldn't think clearly enough to decide who of many I should phone or text for prayer support. Then I gave up and told God that I trusted Him and placed Graeme's life in his hands. He is the only support either of us really need. Into my mind came the verse:

Be still, and know that I am God… (Psalm 46:10)

I relaxed, took slow deep breaths to reduce my racing heart-beats and settled down to rest. Richard was home by 1 a.m., leaving Graeme in hospital for an overnight stay.

Next day, after a toe to groin ultrasound, no DVT was found. Praise the Lord. They could give us no conclusive explanation for the extreme swelling of his ankle except that 'it is related to the chemotherapy'. At least DVT is eliminated as the cause.

Saturday 16 March 2013

> 'Then Jesus said to his disciples: "Therefore I tell you, do not worry about your life, what you will eat; or about your body, what you will wear. Life is more than food, and the body more than clothes."' (Luke 12:22-23)
>
> Many things will try to steal your gaze away from your

God. Worry, materialism, greed, the pervading doctrine of 'self'…are just a few of these things. But we don't have to let them. I want to encourage us all to be content with what we have. We can trust our loving Heavenly Father. It might not work out how we want or how we think it should but, when we live life honouring God, it will work out how He has planned. (Steve McCracken)

Shirley – While in the process of sending out a very overdue email update to our many online friends, I was reminded that in becoming bogged down in our series of health problems I had neglected to give thanks for some of the highlights along the way.

In late January Graeme and I had a quick holiday in Dunedin with my brother and sister-in-law and their family, soaking up the comfort of being amongst people with a shared history who accept you unconditionally. It was a form of healing for us both. Besides having a lot of fun and a few belly laughs, they were very accommodating – letting me doze off and recover between excursions to the beach and countryside.

We've also managed to accept a surprising number of invitations to weddings, birthdays and other special occasions. 'Surprising' because it often came down to making a decision on the day based on how I was feeling. I usually made the effort and was rewarded with some thoroughly enjoyable outings.

There have also been many God moments when the truth from His word springs out from pages of books I feel compelled to pick up – usually when I am most in need of them. And on a down day I will hear a notification on my mobile that I have mail and there will be a text from Michelle; or the phone will go and it will be a friend inviting me out for coffee (and if I'm not up to it, bringing takeaways). Often Graeme will surprise me with an early return from work or arrive with some special treat he knows I will appreciate. All these things remind me that I am loved and that I am not alone.

Along the way, we have become 'experts' on chemotherapy. It's probably fair to say that we all know of at least one person who has been diagnosed with cancer (current scary statistics in New Zealand are that one in three of us will have some form of it) and have heard some hair-raising stories. Most of us would also assume that treatment and side effects are the same for everyone. But surprise, surprise, what we quickly discovered is that no two people are the same. All of us being treated in the oncology room can be on different treatments and quite diverse journeys; it means we don't have to justify treatments and the decisions we've made.

Graeme ~ Who could have foreseen those last nine months? Certainly we all experience our share of unpredictables in life, but usually they come in manageable waves – not a tsunami. There were many times when we felt as if we were drowning, but prayer and our unshakable belief that we were in God's hands kept us afloat.

Further to Shirley's comments regarding the different reactions to chemotherapy, I am amazed at my own naivety at the time; I had taken the tablet option because 'it should be easier.' Probably the reality was exacerbated by the fact that I had been so blasé and had unrealistic expectations, so I was unprepared for the severity of my extreme reactions. Initially, Oncology encouraged me to keep going but ultimately agreed that it was not for me and they would not prescribe it again. To be brutally honest, those weeks of taking chemotherapy medication were probably the worst weeks of my life.

Monday 25 March 2013

He restores my soul. He guides me in the paths of righteousness for his name's sake. Even though I walk through the valley of the shadow of death, I will fear no evil, for you are with me; your rod and your staff, they comfort me. (Psalm 23:3-4)

These [trials] have come so that your faith – of greater worth than gold, which perishes even though refined by fire – may be proved genuine and may result in praise, glory and honour when Jesus Christ is revealed. (1 Peter 1:7)

Shirley – This morning I had an appointment with the massage therapist, who is a very experienced practitioner. But you would think someone in this position would understand the power of positive thinking and be careful not to use negative language. I shuddered when, as we were discussing a plan for my ongoing treatment, she inserted the words: 'for the time you have left'. Reminds me that medical practitioners generally don't understand the God aspect.

Back to the oncologist later in the morning. My tumour marker blood test result is way down, Praise the Lord. He also checked out a few reflexes in my knees, ankles and feet. All were in good working order, to which he said, 'So that means your motor nerves are normal, the numbness and pins and needles is caused by the chemotherapy' – no blockage in the brain, spine or leg pathways. That is all wonderful news.

An email was waiting from Julie telling me that she recently had this 'Horrible, really horrible dream. Horrible! There was all this blood and disgusting stuff.' When she woke up and told her husband he asked her what the horrible stuff was. She said, 'God showed me it was all the ugly cancerous growth that has come out of Shirley.' How graphic is that? It's almost too much to take in, so many amazing things that God shows people.

And then in the afternoon I had a phone call from a friend whose attitude is typical of many Christians who aren't comfortable with our interpretation of the truth about healing. Referring to our weekend away the comment was, 'It's nice to do that while you can.' Well-intentioned I'm sure, but we aren't on the same page and comments like this potentially undermine our faith. But my equilibrium returned and I smiled to myself when I recalled a colleague who had a saying, 'God save me from people with good intentions.'

Sunday 31 March 2013

> Let us then approach the throne of grace with confidence, so that we may receive mercy and find grace to help us in our time of need. (Hebrews 4:16)

> I was always trying to do something and leave God out of the loop. But God will never let us succeed without Him. If He did, we would take all the credit. I learned to pray for what I needed and allowed God to provide it His way, in His timing. When I did, I entered into His rest. (Joyce Meyer, source unknown)

Shirley – Today is Easter Sunday and we need no reminder to celebrate Jesus' resurrection – His saving grace and power.

This morning at church, another well-meaning Christian friend noted that I was looking 'very well… at this stage.' Ugh. Makes us question how much real support there is here for our faith and belief in healing. We wonder if the majority are just mouthing platitudes when they actually believe I am putting on a brave face while I make funeral arrangements.

Graeme ~ There was rarely a day when we didn't receive emails, cards or phone calls from well-wishers. We were grateful for every one of them and never questioned their motivation and good intent. Sometimes it seemed that their opinion conflicted with our own and other times it reinforced our resolve. Either way, we knew it was more important for us to be true to what we believed and not be swayed by others' opinions.

Do we hear what we want to hear? See what we want to see? Believe what we want to believe? Probably a little of each at some point in our lives, and maybe those small self-deceptions are what keep us going until we can hear, see and believe without prevarication. All I can say with conviction is that, for me, to believe is to breathe and I cannot live my life without the guiding light of my Lord. So if I choose to believe that messages sent by others are God speaking through them, then I will gladly take any comfort I can from them and focus on the message not the messenger.

Tuesday 2 April 2013

> 'For God did not give us a spirit of timidity, but a spirit of power, of love and of self-discipline.' (2 Timothy 1:7)
> Renew your mind daily. In order to improve your life you need to change two things:
> Your thought processes: people who are out of shape mentally can fall victim to ideas and systems that are destructive to the human spirit. They grow dependent on the opinions of others. Set a lifelong pursuit of the growth of the mind.

> Your expectations: Faith produces excitement, commitment, energy – characteristics that help you achieve success. Raise your expectation level and bring it into alignment with God's promises – 'Therefore, I tell you, whatever you ask for in prayer, believe that you have received it, and it will be yours.' (Mark 11:24) (*Word for Today*)

Shirley – By this time I have been collecting them for so long that I have a deep reservoir of nourishing words I can immerse myself in whenever I needed sustenance. I recognise the importance for me to use uplifting words and thoughts and surround myself with positive people. I am attempting to drown out any negative words or thoughts and stay focused and strong in my faith. I am drowning in His words.

Thursday 4 April 2013

Shirley – Have once again asked God to show me if my belief regarding healing is wrong. It is confusing when I want to feel completely healed but cannot deny the fact that I'm still experiencing severe peripheral neuropathy. I have received so many words of prophecy and the power and strength of God's Word all supporting our own faith. I guess what I am saying is that it would be wonderful to have all my strength back so I can get going again. But I know in my heart that God wants me to give Him more of my time.

> What will it take for you to come to that settled place where the central desire of your life is, 'God I just want more of you.' (*Word for Today*)

Saturday 6 April 2013

Shirley – I keep googling all about Vinorelbine and chemotherapy-induced peripheral neuropathy in an attempt to reassure myself, but it's probably having the opposite effect. Reversible and irreversible is unknown – you just take your chances. No one warns you how serious it is and it's taken for granted in a clinical sort of way. There's no 'sorry that the poison we gave you has destroyed your nerves and by the way they may, or may not, grow again'. Statistically you have a 30 percent chance of this happening. Doctors, in general, give no information, support or guidance on how to build up the immune system again in order for your body to fight off all that poison. If it wasn't for our own initiatives, we'd probably still be ill. No information about what to eat or natural remedies to take to help in the restorative process. The system really fails us on these important points.

Michelle and Dale are away for the weekend and left their new kitten here to destroy our net curtains and indoor plants. All in all he's quite a placid little kitty, just goes nuts at times and does the weirdest manoeuvres – especially on the kitchen tiles with u-turns and uncontrolled sliding while chasing a ball of tinfoil. So funny! We are all pretty sold on him but I wouldn't be prepared to go through all the carnage razor sharp claws create if we were to get a cat of our own. Besides, it's more about the inconvenience (as M and D are experiencing) when we go away.

Saturday 13 April 2013

Shirley – Looking back over my notes, I'm not aware of having written two of the three significant experiences that happened during August last year. The first two happened while I was driving down to Albany, literally crying to the Lord about my deepest concerns:

1. After much prayer I broached a big question to God: If I'm not healed, and die of this cancer as medically predicted, I can't bear to think my children may turn against you and say: 'If God didn't hear Mum's prayers, and respond to all the others who prayed for her to be healed, He obviously doesn't care. What's the point in trusting and believing in Him?' My soul was in agony. Then I very clearly heard the words: 'You can trust me with your children.' Simple but profound, and it immediately put my heart at ease. Thank you Lord – He knows that, above all, my prayer would be that our children are drawn closer to Him through all of this and become very strong in their faith.
2. I was struck with the awkwardness I would feel when facing the husbands of three women I knew who have recently died from cancer. They had every right to question the fact that I had been healed and their wives had not. Why me? Why was I so special? Why did God save one and not the others? Once again, I heard a very clear voice say: 'It's not about you. It's by my grace.'
3. I was deeply concerned for the many others who believe I will be healed. They have been praying on my behalf, and some are fasting and having dreams. How would they react if I were to die? Then I was reminded about the response I received from a friend when I posed the same question to her: 'You are doing us all a favour – giving us a reason to come closer to the Master ourselves. Don't worry about the time and energy expended on your behalf, you are ushering us into heaven's courts and we will all thank

you for that in the long run. Besides, it is our choice to believe and pray.'

So yet again, God demonstrated that when I hand over all my cares and woes to Him, He listens and always reassures me. I am reminded to have faith in His love and compassion.

Sunday 14 April 2013

Shirley ~ Last night Graeme and I were discussing the reactions to our 'healing journey' we are observing. Sure, we have many wonderful prayer supporters, but how many really believe with us that not only is God able to heal but that He is willing to do it today? We started counting friends who we knew were totally behind us in trusting God's word: 'by his wounds we are healed.' (Isaiah 53:5) We felt somewhat isolated. Certainly many at our church are very hesitant to step out and really believe with us but, praise the Lord, there are also a good handful that are. It reminded us of the prophet Elijah who cried out to God saying, 'I'm the only person left who trusts you.' Well, fortunately for us that's not quite the case.

Today a couple invited us to visit them before they return to overseas ministry later this week. What a most rewarding surprise when we discovered that these dear folk from a conservative Brethren background have frequently been witnessing healing and other spiritual miracles first-hand. We had such an encouraging discussion and prayer time. God is certainly moving among His people. It was wonderfully reassuring after last night's chat.

Monday 15 April 2013

Shirley ~ God, You know my heart. After reading Mary Neal's book *To Heaven and Back* I am euphoric about the prospect of being with you. There is no fear or hesitation about making that last journey and crossing over to be with you. And I am overjoyed at the thought of being reunited with my mum. My dilemma, God, is that I have this inner conviction that my work here on earth isn't done. My place for now is here helping the many hurting people I come into contact with. Father, I am open before you. I once again submit myself to you. Thank you for your amazing love.

And then I sat down and read this (Paul's extraordinary prayer in Ephesians):

> For this reason I kneel before the Father, from whom his whole family in heaven and on earth derives its name. I pray that out of his glorious riches he may strengthen you with power through his Spirit in your inner being, so that Christ may dwell in your hearts through faith. And I pray that you, being rooted and established in love, may have power, together with all the saints, to grasp how wide and long and high and deep is the love of Christ, and to know this love that surpasses knowledge – that you may be filled to the measure of all the fullness of God. Now to him who is able to do immeasurably more than all we ask or imagine, according to his power that is at work within us, to him be glory in the church and in Christ Jesus throughout all generations, for ever and ever! Amen. (Ephesians 3:14-21)

Thursday 18 April 2013

Shirley – Some morsels of wisdom I have been collecting to nourish my soul:

> The mouth of the righteous is a fountain of life... (Proverbs 10:11)

> The tongue of the righteous is choice silver... (Proverbs 10:20)

> The lips of the righteous nourish many... (Proverbs 10:21)

> Your commands make me wiser than my enemies... (Psalm 119:98)

> In Acts 3:6, Peter cries out to a lame man, 'Silver or gold I do not have, but what I have I give you. In the name of Jesus Christ of Nazareth, walk.' The Bible tells us that as Peter took a hold of the man's hands and lifted him, instantly his feet and ankles became strong. (Steve McCracken)

CHAPTER 11

Time Out

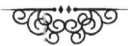

Saturday 20 – Sunday 28 April 2013

Shirley – Some timeout and the pleasure of each other's company in a different environment was just what we needed to restore some balance. It is often not until you stand back from a situation that you can view it more clearly, and although we both knew we had been living with a huge amount of stress, the enormity of it hit us in hindsight and we realised that we had been staggering under a weight that had almost crushed us. For a time it seemed that we had taken leave of cancer and escaped – back to just us and God without that fourth entity hovering and constantly intruding.

We were like a couple of carefree honeymooners – oohing and aahing at the sights as we visited Queenstown and Christchurch and marvelling at nature's spectacular display of autumn foliage. We enjoyed amazing hospitality, and despite the sad glimpses of post-earthquake Christchurch, loved the quirky new architecture and innovative temporary retail strip. I am reminded to give thanks that after so many years together Graeme and I still take pleasure in each other's company.

Wednesday 1 May 2013

'He restores me' – If I ever asked 'Why?' – THIS is the answer: 'The Lord is my shepherd, I shall not be in want. He makes me lie down in green pastures, he leads me beside quiet waters, he restores my soul.' (Psalm 23:1-3a)

Many of us need this today; we need our souls restored. We are spiritual beings living in human bodies in a relational world that is broken and hurting. Our soul affects us greatly and many times we don't know how to handle it.

Is there a quick-fix pill that solves all our problems? I don't think so but I believe there are many things we can do to help us, including prayer, rest, meditation on the Word, talking to someone, getting a hobby, getting a vision, seeing a doctor, getting some exercise and the list goes on. Is there one essential ingredient regardless of the cause or the cure? Yes and we see it clearly here. Psalms says 'HE restores my soul'. We need God, we absolutely do. We can try as hard as we like and many times it will end in deeper frustration. We need God and we need to allow Him to restore us. He may do this supernaturally all by Himself but He also may do it by prompting us where to go and what to do. We must be careful not to miss God's restoration because it came in a box we didn't expect. (Steve McCracken)

Julie – Feel very strongly that this message was directed at you:

> He has spoken to me, and he himself has done this. I will walk humbly all my years because of this anguish of my soul. Lord, by such things men live; and my spirit finds life in them too. You restored me to health and let me live. Surely it

was for my benefit that I suffered such anguish. In your love you kept me from the pit of destruction; you have put all my sins behind your back. (Isaiah 38:15-17)

And in relation to what others may think about you being healed or not, I think this aspect of your journey is far more important: How can they have hope if they don't see hope in you? How can they have courage if they don't see courage in you? How can they know Jesus if they don't see Jesus in you?

Thursday 2 May 2013

Shirley – It's so good to be nearly free of all those severe chemotherapy side effects. Graeme and I are almost at the same level of recovery and finding our energy levels slowly returning. For Graeme this means he is able to concentrate on building up his weight and fitness again in preparation for the reversal operation. Although I've still got numbish feet and weakish hands and knees, they're all becoming more functional now, which is a good indication that the nerves are repairing.

This is how a new baby must feel – wriggling its hands and toes, delighting in its movement and getting stronger day by day as muscles lose their flabbiness. It's like a total rejuvenation – being given a new life with a restored body, mind and soul – it's an amazing feeling.

Wednesday 8 May 2013

'Along unfamiliar paths I will guide them…' (Isaiah 42:16)
Change forces us out of our comfort zone and into the discomfort of the unfamiliar. And while it can turn your world

upside down, it makes you face your greatest fears and deal with the things that steal your joy, peace, and confidence. Change can be your friend or foe, depending on how you use it. Running away turns it into an enemy; embracing and learning from it makes it one of your greatest allies.

When you are facing the unknown, instead of automatically going into resistance mode, 'Fix your eyes on what lies before you... stay on the safe path.' (Proverbs 4:25-26 NLT) Ask yourself: What is God trying to teach me? How can I become stronger and wiser? What opportunities does it hold? You don't have to fear what lies ahead. 'Along unfamiliar paths I will guide them; I will turn the darkness into light before them and make the rough places smooth... I will not forsake them.' God never closes a door without opening another one – but you must be willing to walk through. (*Word for Today*)

Shirley – When I read the *Word for Today* it really made me think about the changes I have experienced in my life while on this prolonged cancer journey. I took stock of my reaction to each aspect of my treatment and how it had forced me to think, act, behave and live in a different way in order to deal with the adjustments it was necessary to make. I would like to think that (if not always immediately) I managed to find some positive within each experience, and hopefully it has made me a stronger person. Surely the best thing to have come out of this is having the time and space to be more reflective; to appreciate the simple things in life and to never ever take the people and things I value for granted. But by far and away my greatest blessing has been the deepening relationship I have with God. He has spoken to me when I needed words; sent messengers when I felt alone; comforted me when I was in pain; reassured me when I had doubts; loved me unconditionally when I ranted and raved; and carried me when I was weak. I now completely understand that my relationship with God is as essential to me as breathing. And more importantly, I am ready to be with Him whenever He asks.

Thursday 9 May 2013

Shirley ~ Yay! I am still going strong and get to celebrate another birthday. Sixty-one years old (words look better than all those stark numerals) and most days feeling every minute of them. But I do find it amusing that under normal circumstances I would not be boasting about it; more likely rushing off to the hairdressers to get the grey covered after rummaging through my wardrobe to find something that, if not entirely slimming, was at least flattering.

Many cards and messages, but this one from a friend moved me to tears:

> God gave a gift to the world when you were born. It would be a privilege to be this person: a person who loves and cares, who sees another's need and fills it, who encourages and lifts people up, who spends energy on others rather than herself, who touches each life she enters and makes a difference in the world. May the love you have shown to others return to you multiplied. Happy Birthday. Have an awesome birthday today and wonderful year ahead. With love and prayers.

And yes, I had a fabulous day surrounded by my wonderful family, deluged with thoughtful gifts and being extravagantly spoilt.

Friday 10 May 2013

Shirley ~ It seems crazy that again I've had unintended discouraging comments from other Christians – people you would rightfully expect to support us in building up our faith and hope. So discouraging to hear someone say, 'It's great that you are feeling better just now' or 'I heard that you were looking very good at the moment.' I even heard that folk we are meeting with from our previous church are really looking forward to seeing me. I felt like Exhibit A. But God has reminded me that 'it's not about you, it's by my grace,' and I try not to let it affect me.

I'm learning that all these examples are not personal and not specifically aimed at my journey with cancer – the comments unfortunately reflect either a lack of relationship with God or a limited understanding and trust in God's almighty power. We are so excited that one day we can show that 'terminal cancer' isn't necessarily terminal to God.

Friday 24 May 2013

Shirley ~ I think that one of the toughest challenges as a Christian is attempting to interpret God's will. We want to be obedient but sometimes have difficulty following His instructions – the issue is whether we have understood clearly or heard what we wanted to hear. My constant dilemma has been conflicting messages. I believe that God can heal me but I do not know in my heart if this is what He considers the best outcome for my eternal soul. However, I do know that I surrender to His will.

And after a period of quiet reflection about how I will know God's will, I picked up a book and as per usual the appropriate message popped up:

Do not conform any longer to the pattern of this world, but be transformed by the renewing of your mind. Then you will be able to test and to approve what God's will is – His good, pleasing and perfect will. (Romans 12:2)

But just in case His will is for me to be healed, I am collecting verses that are filled with His promises. These are my favourite verses regarding healing:

Jesus healed all who came to Him: 'Many followed him, and he healed all their sick.' (Matthew 12:15) 'and all who touched him were healed.' (Matthew 14:36) 'and the people all tried to touch him, because power was coming from him and healing them all.' (Luke 6:19) 'I tell you the truth, my Father will give you whatever you ask in my name.' (John 16:23)

Friday 31 May 2013

The LORD is my rock, my fortress and my deliverer; my God is my rock, in whom I take refuge, my shield and the horn of my salvation. He is my stronghold, my refuge and my saviour – from violent men you save me. I call to the LORD, who is worthy of praise, and I am saved from my enemies. (2 Samuel 22:2-4)

Shirley – 'Violent men and enemies' don't figure in my life but it struck me that God saves/protects me from the emotional toll that comes with deflecting opinions from people – in the medical profession particularly – who aren't coming from the same God perspective as us. The Lord certainly is my rock. I could of course relate the 'violence' to the harsh chemicals which were used to attack damaged organs in my body (the temple of my soul?).

Tuesday 4 June 2013

> Faith is a law and we operate in it with our words, either to our benefit or our destruction… 'The tongue of the wise brings healing.' (Proverbs 12:18) (Mark Brazee in *365 Days of Healing*)

Shirley ~ My prayer: 'Lord, you have given me SO MANY promises in your Word regarding hope, healing and return to full health. Father, I'm open to you, you know that. But I have never had confirmation and peace from you that this cancer prognosis spells the end of my life here on earth. Quite the contrary. So Lord, I give to you my niggly back, I give to you what seems like numbness starting to creep up my legs from my already partially numb feet. Lord, I'm trusting you alone. I love you, Lord, and I want your perfect will in my life. I have no doubt in my mind regarding your healing power and willingness to heal me. Show me, Lord, please.'

> And if the Spirit of him, who raised Jesus from the dead, is living in you, he who raised Christ from the dead will also give life to your mortal bodies through his Spirit, who lives in you. (Romans 8:11)

Wednesday 5 June 2013

Shirley ~ Didn't sleep too well last night. Just wondering what

God is up to. Have I read Him wrong? Yet I trust God's Word totally to heal me. I really do. It's not blind faith. It's real faith based on His Word. My wonderful understanding husband knows the confusion constantly raging in my mind. This morning he left these words of encouragement for me knowing that God would use them to raise me up:

'Blessed is she who has believed that what the Lord has said to her will be accomplished!' (Luke 1:45) What a powerful testimony – one that we too can have.

You might be facing an apparent giant this year. But I declare 'with God, all things are possible!' (Matthew 19:26) Your giant can be defeated this year. God does not lie. God always completes what He starts.

So let's walk with Him. Let's believe in His Word and His promises to us. Let's set our minds and hearts to staying in faith no matter what. This is a year of dreams turning into realities…and faith is essential. (Steve McCracken)

And the prayer offered in faith will make the sick person well; the Lord will raise them up. (James 5:15)

A man wrote, 'Last year doctors discovered a cancerous tumour on my bladder and immediately arranged surgery. I knew Jesus was the best doctor in the world, so I prayed for Him to touch me and I believed that I was healed. When I told the doctors, they looked at me and said nothing in case it would discourage me but when they performed the surgery, they found there wasn't a trace of cancer – I was completely whole.' This man is now perfectly healthy and rejoicing in the Lord. (Willie Baptiste Florian in Fiji)

Thursday 6 June 2013

Shirley ~ Two nights ago we prayed, 'Father, please show us if I should have a CT scan as the oncologist wants.' I'm not keen to have one because my body doesn't need another load of radiation. What do I do? Seriously, how will God answer that prayer? Well, today I was talking with a friend in a totally different context and she mentioned that the doctor wanted her to have an amniocentesis in pregnancy because of her older age. She chose not to because she wouldn't be willing to follow through and have an abortion if the foetus was found to have Down's Syndrome. Coincidentally, I had been in the same predicament with our two children.

Immediately, I related this situation back to the similarities of my current dilemma and it gave me a clearer perspective. Quite simply, if the results from a CT scan were bad, I'm not willing to follow through and have any further chemotherapy treatment. The recent course of treatment I endured was reportedly 'thrashing you with the hardest we've got'. If that treatment didn't work, why would I want to go through that horror again with similar ineffective results? So that helps clarify my decision.

The only other consideration is having a CT scan to show that God has healed me so that we can confidently speak out. That would be wonderful, but is this God's timing to announce to the world His amazing grace in my life?

> Being fully persuaded that God had power to do what he had promised. (Romans 4:21)

Friday 7 June 2013

> Praise the Lord ... who crowns you with love and compassion, who satisfies your desires with good things so that your youth is renewed like the eagle's. (Psalm 103:1,4-5)

Shirley ~ It was our usual Friday morning prayer for our families today. I've been meeting with other Christians on a weekly basis for so many years (in Auckland and now Orewa) and have experienced many blessings. I am so grateful for their prayers for my health and wholeness, and more specifically today, for the healing of my side pain, diaphragm and back (caused by pleurodesis).

More study and reflection on knowing God's will. God is teaching us more and more in the area of praying for healing. The 'if it is your will' postscript somehow gets added by so many to give God (and the person praying?) a cop out. Our God does not need a cop out.

> The thief comes only to steal and kill and destroy; I have come that they may have life, and have it to the full. (John 10:10)

Tuesday 18 June 2013

Shirley ~ Had an appointment with the oncologist yesterday. He is satisfied that he can't identify any obvious signs of cancer. However, although it isn't an indicator in itself, the tumour marker blood test result was slightly raised. But it would be of concern if the next result (in six weeks) showed a similar trend.

I felt okay initially but as the day progressed the doubts started creeping in and I felt discouraged. I asked God for reassurance and amazingly once again He gave me peace.

I tell you the truth, if you have faith as small as a mustard seed, you can say to this mountain, 'Move from here to there' and it will move. Nothing will be impossible for you. (Matthew 17:20-21)

God is amazing. Today He arranged for two people to speak faith to me using the same verse:

Now faith is being sure of what we hope for and certain of what we do not see. (Hebrews 11:1)

Wednesday 19 – Saturday 22 June 2013

Shirley – Graeme and I attended the Kingdom Come three-and-a-half-day conference. The two speakers were Randy Clark and Chris Gore from Bethel Church in Redding, California. Some snippets and gems:

Faith is like using God's muscle – it's all of Him through all of me. We are not there to partner with a person's problem but to partner with the answer – don't be impressed by the problem, be impressed by the answer – let the answer become bigger than the problem. Grace is free but the kingdom will cost you everything. Faith is a by-product of looking into the eyes of Jesus Christ. Darkness is the absence of light – we need to feel the light of Jesus, not the darkness around us. Christianity is often reduced to a gospel of salvation only.

> How we deal with disappointments now is how we will cope with tomorrow. When some aren't healed, the burden isn't ours – when some are healed, the glory is His.

And this particularly resonates:

> Why don't people pray for healing? They have an intellectual approach and need an answer why God doesn't heal some. Pride – they don't want to look like failures. It hurts – there's emotional pain for those healing and praying if there is no healing. Apart from the love of God we would quit. Healing is in the cross: 'If anyone would come after me, he must deny himself and take up his cross daily and follow me.' (Luke 9:23) If healing doesn't happen, you will quit if you don't have total love of God and trust Him even though healing hasn't happened. Offer a sacrifice of praise in the midst of suffering and disappointments.

> for I am the LORD, who heals you. (Exodus 15:26)

> The power of humility: Having full access to God should never bring pride. Without God we can do nothing. We need to stay a novice, totally dependent on Him. When we become self-sufficient, we start leaving God out. Stay humble and always give God the glory. If you are in a church that isn't open to healing and miracles, have a servant attitude. Serve without changing your core convictions.

> Healing: There is no formula for healing. God doesn't do the same for everyone.

Monday 24 June 2013

Shirley – It's so good to be nearly free of all the severe chemotherapy side effects and to have so much more energy. I've still got the numbish feet and weakish hands and knees from the peripheral neuropathy but nerves must be growing back as they're becoming more functional. I can walk now without being afraid I might fall over. I was told it could take six to twelve months for the nerve damage to repair, if it is reversible, so I'm grateful for the good progress so far. It's also fantastic to have my brain back out of a fog – although I must admit it was quite useful at times using that excuse.

I still have quite a bit of diaphragm pain from the pleurodesis. The oncologist has suggested a CT scan, but I've made it clear that I am in no hurry to have another large shot of radiation. I also suspect that more chemotherapy would be the order if he wasn't happy with the result – as if!

But hey, we are very grateful to God for His compassion towards us, for His saving grace and power. Why us? That's not the point – it is God's grace to us. It is for God to receive all the glory. He wants to be a testimony through our lives.

And as if God hasn't given me enough to celebrate lately, we are filled with joy and anticipation about our expected grandchild due in two months' time. Michelle and Dale shared their wonderful news with us in January but were understandably reluctant to make it too public until she was further advanced – she is now sporting a very cute little 'preggie' bump. They are looking forward to a big change in their lives, and I give thanks that I can be here to share this joyous time with all my family.

He has spoken to me, and he himself has done this. I will walk humbly all my years because of this anguish of my soul. Lord, by such things men live; and my spirit finds life in them too. You restored me to health and let me live. Surely it was for my benefit that I suffered such anguish. In your love you kept me from the pit of destruction; you have put all my sins behind your back. (Isaiah 38:15-17)

Graeme – Once I stopped chemotherapy in early March, my recovery was remarkable. From looking like a scarecrow, with wiry hair and peeling hands and feet, I regained most of my weight and energy levels within a couple of months. In fact, after the initial period following surgery, I had only four days off work (coping with the worst of my reaction to all that poison seeping through my system).

Once again I was wracked with guilt. My symptoms, while decidedly unpleasant, were comparatively short-lived and I had no lingering side effects, while Shirley's suffering was at times debilitating and her recovery much more prolonged.

Wednesday 26 June 2013

Shirley – From the strange reactions I get, it seems prudent to not expect excitement from many Christians about the wonderful healing God is doing in my body. It's been my choice (made in total accord with Graeme) to stick out our necks and publicly proclaim our belief that God will heal me. But it can be emotionally draining when confronted with doubt.

Attempt great things for God and expect great things from

God. When human wisdom and ability won't take you a step further, faith will, because faith holds the hand of God. And 'with God all things are possible' (Matthew 19:26). Just make sure you are acting in faith and not presumption.

Obstacles and opposition are inevitable; they are part of the journey. But you must not allow them to make you doubt God and what He's called you to do.

'Yet he did not waver through unbelief regarding the promise of God, but was strengthened in his faith and gave glory to God, being fully persuaded that God had the power to do what he had promised.' (Romans 4:20-21) (William Carey)

Friday 28 June 2013

Shirley ~ We are in God's hands – what better place could there be? I see this time now as letting my body (and mind) recover from all the trauma of the last year. It would be so easy to get back on the bandwagon and go for it but this new (wiser?) Shirley is prepared to choose more carefully where I place my time and energy and make haste slowly.

Julie ~ As always, praying for you. Not only for healing but also for courage to face each new day and new challenge; patience and trust that He has a much bigger plan of which you are a part; and the knowledge and belief that you are precious to Him.

Thursday 11 July 2013

Be still, and know that I am God; I will be exalted among the nations, I will be exalted in the earth. (Psalm 46:10)

Shirley – Have had a heavy cold for over a week now and am on antibiotics. First cold since having the pleurodesis procedure performed last year. I have been coughing and coughing – it sounds so chesty – and occasionally a small 'plug' (according to the GP) comes up. Thinking that a bit more of that would be a great relief, we asked for it at our prayer time this morning and from that time it felt as if my lungs had been cleared. Thank you, Lord.

Thursday 18 July 2013

Shirley – Guess what? I've spent the last week non-stop coughing and coughing. It's reached the point where I am coughing so much every day that I am exhausted. So much so that today, after thanking God for answering last week's prayer, I asked that the excessive mucous would be dried up in my lungs. I actually found this sequence quite amusing and was reminded to be careful how I phrased my requests in future. Wow, again, what an amazing God. First day that I haven't spent bent in half coughing myself crazy.

If that's not good enough, get this: the last few days I've had sharp pains in my lumbar spine, slightly restricting my movements. My mind goes straight to the cancer diagnosis. Together with the persistent coughing, my mind has been working overtime – 'God, what is going on here? I'm totally trusting you for healing. I'm believing your Word.' Again I've had that night panic and sick feeling. Again I've resisted Satan's lies and claimed God's power in my life. So more prayer today, anointing with oil, and I've been released from the pain. My heart is full of praise to our wonderful loving Heavenly Father.

Saturday 20 July 2013

Shirley ~ The process of documenting the conundrum presented by my total belief that God will heal me, and the visible evidence that this is not happening, helps me to see my way back on track and strengthens my resolve. When I feel under attack or I'm in the presence of someone who is patronisingly saying words of encouragement while we both know they think I am kidding myself, I am at a loss for words. So the following are my thoughts about the way some people are chipping away at my faith with their negativity:

When we are faced with a crisis, or perhaps a life/death situation like us, we need to know that we can trust God and His Word without doubting. Our faith needs to grow strong. But if we have been basing our study of God's Word primarily on academia and scholarly theories it is difficult, when we are under pressure, to discern the truth in Scripture. What can we take literally? Miracles and truths previously considered in the context of Bible times only add to our confusion, or we miss the point and the blessing that God has for us TODAY. When the academic side is overemphasised, personal truth is diminished.

> 'The tongue has the power of life and death, and those who love it will eat its fruit.' (Proverbs 18:21)
>
> Your words either work for you or against you. The old saying, 'You'll eat your words,' is not a meaningless cliché, it's the truth. 'They cried out to the LORD in their trouble, and he saved them out of their distresses. He sent his word and healed them...' (Psalm 107:19-20 NKJV) God's Word is the medicine that heals us. So what God has to say about the issue must be what you have to say about it too, otherwise

you're contradicting Him and disconnecting yourself from the source of all blessing. If you're wise, you will surround yourself with like-minded people who speak God's Word into your life, and limit your time with those who have no interest in it. If you want to grow the right kind of fruit, you must have the right climate. And the words you speak (and listen to) determine the climate of your life, the direction in which it goes, and the results you get. (*Word for Today*)

Thursday 25 July 2013

The LORD would speak to Moses face to face, as one speaks to a friend… (Exodus 33:11)

Shirley – I can't remember where I heard this but it really hit home: Knowing that God is always with us does not constitute an intimate relationship – spending dedicated, regular, one-on-one time with Him does.

It occurred to me that because God is so elevated (in terms of being our Lord) we communicate with Him in stilted ways. We either follow some formalised prayer or scripture or speak in an unnatural jargonistic formula. And it's all pretty much one-sided. If we were to consider God as a person we want to develop an intimate relationship with, we would know that it is not about to happen unless we take the time to get to know Him. Deep and meaningful friendships are built on mutual trust and respect; being available to each other when needed; having regular open communication; showing you care in as many ways as possible; sharing your innermost thoughts; inviting feedback and actively listening. A true friendship is one that offers unconditional love – has hope but no expectations.

Monday 29 July 2013

Shirley – To the oncologist again today – visit number…? I've lost count. Discouraging news – I was aghast to be told that the blood tumour marker test results are higher. Also it appears that the adenocarcinoma on my left breast may be reappearing. The oncologist's projected plan for my future was very palliative and about 'giving you time'. We came away feeling so discouraged that I spent the rest of the day questioning all the words of healing and encouragement I've been given. My faith feels rock-bottom. I feel at the end of it. Can God forgive all that? It is a very difficult time for us both.

CHAPTER 12

Rays of Light

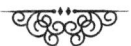

Tuesday 30 July 2013

Shirley – We know of a young lady who is going through a major medical issue at the moment. She openly expressed her doubt and fears on Facebook, which gave me the opportunity to interject. I replied saying, 'It's okay that you don't understand all you are going through. And it's true that no one else can really know how you feel – but we do care so much for you. And we can ask God for His peace so you can totally trust HIM. I love the verse that says: "Great is our Lord and mighty in power; his understanding has no limit." (Psalm 147:5) He does listen and He does understand. You are not alone.'

A short while later I was feeling much lighter in spirit and realised that having the opportunity to express myself in order to help someone else had also encouraged me. In my much perkier mood I had a sudden recollection of bits of a song from my grandmother's era that had the refrain: 'Some days are diamonds some days are pearls' – it's a good way to describe the variances of my topsy-turvy life at the moment.

Let your eyes look straight ahead; fix your gaze directly before

Peace in the Storm

you. Make level paths for your feet and take only ways that are firm. (Proverbs 4:25-26)

The implications of this proverb for me are: (a) don't get sidetracked by oncologist's 'medical facts' and others' negativity; (b) put my focus on God's truth and keep it there, no matter what; and (c) trust Him!

Not an easy thing to do – stay firmly on the path. Sometimes I feel as if I have stepped onto an escalator wearing a blindfold, being relentlessly carried along with absolutely no idea where I will end up. Those are the times I rely on God to be my compass and guide.

So after my major 'blah', I need to reconnect with God and totally trust Him – no matter the outcome of this unenviable situation. My challenge is to keep believing I will be healed despite the setbacks and God's seeming non-intervention at this stage.

Wednesday 31 July 2013

'But one thing I do: Forgetting what is behind and straining toward what is ahead, I press on toward the goal to win the prize for which God has called me heavenward in Christ Jesus.' (Philippians 3:13-14)

Live a focused life; forget past failures; have intense anticipation of future success; have a full-on defence. (*Word for Today*)

Shirley ~ Lest we become too complacent, another challenge is thrown before us. Graeme called to say that his visit to Specsavers, to check out an increasing blurring of his right eye over the last two days, resulted in being sent straight to an eye specialist, where he was diagnosed with a retinal tear. It was so acute that he was admitted immediately into Greenlane Eye Clinic where he had laser surgery. Praise the Lord, the treatment was effective.

When Richard and I went to the city, so that one of us could drive him home, Graeme suggested that we attend a local Christian centre. Without this incident we probably wouldn't have thought of going to the meeting.

The speaker talked about deliverance from Satan's clutches. The message was based around the armour of God in the sixth chapter of Ephesians. After the meeting, we were prayed for by a lady who seemed very much in tune with the Lord. After hearing about our situation at the oncologist two days ago, she said that his words of doom and gloom, about 'buying time, terminal management and further chemotherapy' had opened me/us to the spirit of death.

> The tongue has the power of life and death... (Proverbs 18:21)

We were also exposed to spirits of doubt and fear. So we prayed on it and a dark cloud was lifted from us.

The lady claimed healing again for my body. We were impressed that she listened to God and had a real neat anointing in her ministering. She then prayed for Graeme, for wholeness and healing. It was an enormous sense of release for us both. This has all made me realise that the words of death spoken at some medical appointments basically make us give up and think that we are dying. The power of those doom words is so strong but not as strong as God's words of life.

Julie ~ How wonderful. God is on the throne and He had

that lady all ready and prepared for you. That is so much the enemy – having the oncologist send you into a pit of despair, then whacking Graeme with a detached retina. But God came through trumps, didn't He?

Thursday 1 August 2013

Shirley ~ My dad's eighty-ninth birthday today – we are so blessed to have had him with us for so long, and now there is the opportunity for another generation to benefit from his presence in their life. And yet again (as I do now for each special occasion) I give my heartfelt thanks to God that I am here to celebrate yet another year of my dad's life with him. My wonderful father, what a trial we have put him through. Whenever I think of how this dreadful drawn-out saga has been for him, my heart aches – I think it is every parent's nightmare that they will outlive their children.

> I have loved you; therefore I will give men for you, and people for your life. Fear not, for I am with you… (Isaiah 43:4-5 NKJV)

Sunday 4 August, 2013

Shirley ~ During communion, while taking the 'wine' at church today, I was struck with the fact that Jesus' blood was shed for ME. He loves ME so much. It was therefore totally logical that He would also want to heal me because of His great love – 'by his wounds we are healed.' (Isaiah 53:5) Thank you, Lord.

I received a phone call from an extended family member and we discussed the difficult events of the last week. She made an interesting observation: the oncologist was making statements based on statistics and his experience, assuming that the cancer would behave in a certain way, need the usual prescribed treatment and have the usual terminal outcome. None of which takes into consideration my faith in God and His love and power to heal me.

Just the sort of positive reinforcement and encouragement we need to keep both Graeme and me fighting, putting on the whole armour of God, and believing in His Word.

Tuesday 6 August 2013

Shirley ~ Not only does the adenocarcinoma appear to have returned to my left breast but today I noticed that a large swollen gland has appeared above my right collarbone. This is all getting too much. What is going on?

Wednesday 7 August 2013

> We need to be feeding ourselves continually with the truth that can only be found in the Word of God. Louie Giglio said, 'When life hurts the most, the world listens most intently to our message, allowing us to broadcast through our pain the goodness of the One who loves us the most.' It is described as the Megaphone of Hope. (*Word for Today*)

Shirley ~ I know a lot of genuinely concerned people question my choices – the age-old argument that God heals, so I should place myself in His hands and sit back and wait to be healed. But believe me, there is rarely a day when I haven't churned my stomach, swinging first one way and then the other. I have conducted a zillion debates in my head (led by the medical team) and my heart (the Christian team). In attempting to ratify my decisions, I will (for the record) explain why I chose human intervention:

Probably it begins with the fact that I am a nurse. In that capacity, over a lengthy period of time, I developed a healthy respect for doctors and their dedication to healing the sick. And since then, medicine has progressed in leaps and bounds: we have cutting-edge technology, ground-breaking drugs, and highly skilled surgeons with enormous experience in this field. Although I, at no point, took any advice without qualifying it with my own research, it was hard to ignore their 'do or die' prognosis.

And then, how was I to know whether or not I was being led in this direction; that God was speaking through these caring professionals who through Him would eradicate this vile cancer and heal me? Either way it was healing. And maybe going down this road I would meet others along the way that would benefit from my experience.

I didn't know. I still don't know. And at every step of the way I have gone over the same argument. Whenever yet another treatment or operation was on the agenda, and I contemplated the pain and trauma I was setting myself up for, my mind would scream, 'No! Nooooooooo! Please no more!' But my heart would say, 'Be still. Until God indicates otherwise, you are following the path He wants you to take.' And, as always, I would be given the strength and peace to persevere.

For non-Christians it is an equally difficult choice. Recently, while we were in the chemo ward I spoke to a young mother and was moved to tears by her story. She is a solo mum bringing up a 10-year-old daughter on her own. When she was initially diagnosed, she was very clear that she wanted to let nature take its course and not put herself through all this hell to die in the end anyway. But then she looked at her beautiful young daughter and decided that she would do whatever it took to be around long enough to equip the child with the strength and wisdom to carry on without her. No doubt many decisions are based on similar desires – none of us want to think about the pain we would inflict on our loved ones by leaving them (albeit not by choice).

Saturday 10 August 2013

Shirley – Graeme's birthday and another reason to give thanks to God for the time I have with the people I love. Lord, I can never thank you enough for the blessing of my very precious husband.

Today Graeme fasted and prayed, waiting on God regarding my latest developments. During the evening he read from the incident in Exodus 7:8-13 when Moses was before Pharaoh. Moses threw his staff to the ground and it became a snake. Pharaoh's magicians (that is, Satan) could also make this happen. Then Moses' snake turned and ate Pharaoh's snake. Graeme said it is like God was saying to him that it is Satan putting his version of a swollen gland on to me. But we know God's power is greater and He will make it disappear.

Graeme – By now I had become adept at switching off – I knew I couldn't survive, let alone be strong for Shirley, if I gave in to the waking nightmare that was watching my beloved wife slowly but surely lose this battle with cancer. But it is surprising how much we humans can accept if pressure and stress is applied incrementally. The whole family had learnt to cope with each new development in Shirley's saga, to the point where every time something changed, we made a quick adjustment – saw it as the new normal and just got on with it. She behaved as if there was nothing abnormal about having a truckload of medical paraphernalia attached to her wherever she went and simply accepted her own limitations without comment or complaint. We followed suit and continued as if nothing was wrong.

> Peace I leave with you; my peace I give you. I do not give to you as the world gives. Do not let your hearts be troubled and do not be afraid. (John 14:27)

Monday 12 August 2013

Shirley ~ Today the gland is less swollen and the adenocarcinoma skin lesion has shrunk. Hallelujah – another small victory. I do see these as miracles and there have been many.

I was speaking with a friend on the phone and mentioned the two areas of concern. Before I could tell her that the lesion and gland were shrinking, she said, 'This reminds me of Job. Satan put sickness on to Him but God brought him through and healed him.' So perhaps this fight is not just about me – perhaps it's an opportunity for God to demonstrate His power through me.

And maybe it all comes back again to frame of mind. Another friend summarised from a book she was reading by the French philosopher Simone Weil who says that 'the pure love of God means being exactly as grateful for your afflictions as you are for your blessings'. I'm trying – truly I'm trying. I can honestly say that my suffering and afflictions have brought me closer to God, and for that I would without hesitation be prepared to pay any price.

But at times I am weak and it does seem to me that most people draw closer to God when they have afflictions, so I ask, 'Could that be the reason why we have them?' If it is a test of my faith, then I say again, I am prepared to pay the price.

Thursday 15 August 2013

Shirley - Is 'if it is your will' the ultimate cop out in prayer? We ask for what we think/believe is right and leave it to God to decide whether it is right or not. I suggest that means believing God's Word and His many promises, and trusting Him for the ultimate outcome because He is God.

> If you've prayed for the fulfilment of a Bible promise that didn't materialise, you may have wondered, felt disillusioned, or even stopped trusting. What's true is that every promise in the Book intended for you, is yours. God is committed to keeping every promise He has made (Matthew 24:35). But be sure you understand the promise. God is committed to His Word, not to your interpretation of it. (*Word for Today*)

Saturday 17 August 2013

Shirley - This evening, while Graeme and I were talking about future plans – in particular, holidays – I was finding it very difficult to commit myself to anything that far ahead. When he asked me why, the whole issue of CT scans came up, and I admitted that after having far too many that were harbingers of bad news I was scared to have another. I'm finding it very confusing – with all my heart trusting God for healing, yet still terrified of what the scan may show. They are such opposing ideas.

> Very truly I tell you, unless a kernel of wheat falls to the ground and dies, it remains only a single seed. But if it dies, it produces many seeds. (John 12:24)

Sunday 18 August 2013

Shirley ~ Had an awful dream last night that I was lost – stumbling around unable to find my workplace or car. Woke up not feeling good at all. A friend interpreted this as my subconscious dealing with the fact that nothing is familiar any more – my life as I knew it has gone, and I am looking for direction. Well, I'm not about to argue with that.

We decided to accept an invitation to visit a friend's church today. The visiting speaker talked about confusing thoughts in our minds. Ouch, who told him? I confessed to God about being scared, and once again claimed 2 Timothy 1:7.

> For God has not given us a spirit of fear but of power, and of love and of a sound mind. (NKJV)

The speaker then talked about pressing our 'reset button' – re-evaluate our thinking/beliefs and live like we believe it.

This evening Graeme and I decided to formulate a Mission Statement so that we can clarify our head space. At times we have so much emotional and spiritual pressure dealing with medical appointments and forthcoming CT scans that it creates a lot of tension. Especially when opposing belief systems meet.

Graeme ~ This was a rewarding exercise. At the time we formulated this Mission Statement, we were both in a very confused state of mind. Our intent was to reach a space of peace and purpose in our hearts and share that with God. Having an uncluttered understanding of what we wished to achieve, and what we sincerely believed, was enormously helpful and gave us a constructive plan to refer back to whenever we were floundering.

OUR MISSION STATEMENT
- Our desire is that God's name is glorified and exalted through our lives. That the witness of our healing would draw people to Him.
- We believe God's willingness to heal us – through His Word, spiritual revelation and spoken words given to us. We know God is sovereign and we totally trust Him to fulfil His purpose in our lives.
- As in Daniel 3:17-18, even if we are NOT healed this side of heaven, we will still honour, praise and worship God. We don't believe that He is taking us home at this time, but just say that was true, what we are doing is right – believing in our healing and drawing closer to God. It will always be the right thing to do. No matter what the outcome, we desire for our family to give praise to God, not to be disappointed in Him.
- 'My times are in your hands...' (Psalm 31:15) 'All the days ordained for me were written in your book before one of them came to be.' (Psalm 139:16)
- God knows the number of our days, and we trust Him for them. No more, no less.
- We desire to live and be available to encourage and support our children and grandchildren spiritually and physically.
- 'For God did not give us a spirit of timidity [fear], but a spirit of power, of love and of a self-discipline.' (2 Timothy 1:7) We submit ourselves and our family to God's will for

our future so that He is able to fulfil His purpose in us on this earth.

Wednesday 21 August 2013

Shirley ~ Another major milestone and reason to celebrate. Today we became grandparents for the first time. A joy under any circumstances, but increased immeasurably for me by actually being present at the birth of our precious granddaughter, Jasmine Grace McCarter. We praise God for her safe arrival. We are bursting with pride and filled with excitement – can't wait to spend time with her and to watch her grow. We have no doubt that new mum and dad, Michelle and Dale, will be the best parents a little girl could possibly have.

Monday 26 August 2013

Shirley ~ Friends invited us to join them at a healing meeting at their home this evening. Other commitments meant that there were only six of us there, but what we lacked in numbers we made up for in brilliant testimonies, worship and prayer. There were also some remarkable prophecies, such as: 'This sickness is not unto death' and 'I can see you in a teaching role' and 'You will be a shining testimony – God's light shines out from you.'

We very much appreciated so much prayer and support from others who take God at His Word without doubting. Sooooo encouraging. The swollen gland above my right clavicle is still there but won't be for long as it has been well prayed over and 'deactivated'.

And I will do whatever you ask in my name, so that the Father may be glorified in the Son. You may ask me for anything in my name, and I will do it. (John 14:13-14)

Thursday 29 August 2013

Shirley ~ Today is Dale's birthday and we give grateful thanks to our Lord for the blessing of a wonderful son-in-law and Michelle's loving and supportive husband. We have always considered ourselves lucky that our children bring their friends into our home and Dale was a regular visitor long before becoming family. We love having young people around us, and listening to their views challenges our thinking and keeps us on our toes.

Monday 2 September 2013

Shirley ~ Take note: I trimmed the grass along all the concrete edges on our property today (I'll be very disappointed if Graeme doesn't notice when he comes home). It was very tiring at the time but no pain or discomfort afterwards. Must admit to feeling very pleased with myself.

A series of significant contrasts are consistently coming up – light versus darkness, life versus death, trust versus fear, hope versus despair. I would suppose that it is all in keeping with my constant conflict and inability to hold firm when I do make a decision. My biggest issue is questioning my own understanding of God's purpose.

God is light; in him there is no darkness at all. (1 John 1:5)

Tuesday 3 September 2013

Shirley ~ Today Graeme has his stoma reversal operation at Southern Cross Hospital. I do know that it couldn't come soon enough and he can't wait to get his fit and healthy body back into shape. As usual he is remarkably stoic – seeing it all as a slight inconvenience and expecting to be back at work in no time.

It was a relatively short operation compared to the surgery nine months ago. He came out of the operating theatre about 7 p.m. and the surgeon said that everything went very well. By the time I was able to see Graeme, he was already looking bright, pain was under control and he was resigned to taking it easy for a few days. We are very relieved that this latest event is behind us and trust God for full and total healing.

Thursday 5 September 2013

Shirley ~ Received a phone call from my GP. My blood tumour marker test has, over recent months, been sitting around 28, which is within normal limits. Then 12 weeks ago it shot up to 40, then six weeks ago to 60. Now it is 109 – the highest it has been since I first started chemotherapy. Last time, the oncologist said that it was raised because I had a lot of dead cancer cells from the chemo treatment. This time he will be very convinced that it is the cancer coming back in full swing. Apparently the tumour marker is raised by both living and dead cancer cells present in my body.

My first reaction was shock. But I am continuing to believe and trust God will heal me. I am believing that there are copious dead cancer cells being eliminated from my system. I am so grateful that my GP chose to phone me with the results this time. Normally it is the oncologist who tells us the good or bad news, but after our last depressing appointment it is wonderful that he didn't get the opportunity. For this I thank God.

I didn't share any of this with Graeme today, as he isn't feeling too good. But since his condition is as predicted, we are not too concerned. It's uncomfortable, and we will all be very pleased for him when it's over, but meanwhile he just gets on with it.

This journey is sooooo challenging, to say the least. In need of a friend, I sent an email and received an immediate response:

Julie ~ Dear, dear Shirley, What can I say to comfort you? What a terrible shock to get today while your man is recovering from his own operation and needing you to be strong for him.

Yes, Shirley, this journey is veeeeery challenging. First thought – read the lyrics of the song It Is Well With My Soul again. Second thought – give yourself a special treat. Go and eat something your soul is longing for (indulge). Then just sit in your La-Z-Boy chair and surround yourself with music. Immerse yourself in His presence until you get drowsy enough to sleep. Don't let your mind start playing the 'what ifs' and take away your peace.

Dwell in the shadow of the Almighty and let him comfort you, my precious one. Yes, precious – you are very precious in the Lord's sight. You are highly honoured and loved. He will carry you through these dark days and bring you out as pure gold. He is transforming you into His image. So go and sit at His feet and soak in His presence and drink from His cup. Celebrate His love for you.

Friday 6 September 2013

Shirley – We had a beaut time of praise and worship at our regular Friday prayer time this morning; that, I believe, is where it's at. Psalm 103 was highlighted yet again:

> Praise the LORD, my soul; all my inmost being, praise his holy name. Praise the LORD, my soul, and forget not all his benefits – who forgives all your sins and heals all your diseases... (Psalm 103:1-3)

I trust God totally.

Graeme's first day after the operation was great, but alas, as we had been warned, it was the calm before the storm, and the last three days and nights he was up and down to the toilet every ten minutes, vomiting, very high blood pressure. He's very tired.

But we are pleased to be able to confirm the surgeon's prediction that Graeme should come through this 'good'. In fact, we were very amused when the surgeon ascribed his confidence to the fact that Graeme was 'young and fit.' Today Graeme finally started tolerating a small amount of soft food. Progress will apparently take weeks, months, and sometimes two to three years, before a new normal is attained. One would think that joining up a couple of bits of bowel would be straightforward, but apparently the body has a lot of relearning to do.

I finally told Graeme about the raised blood tumour marker result this afternoon. Later I went for a walk in the sun outside the hospital, talking to the Lord and telling Him that I love and trust Him and I only want His best for my life.

Graeme ~ All my own woes were forgotten when Shirley sat down by my hospital bed and told me the results of her blood tumour marker test. This day is another that is imprinted on my memory forever. I was stunned, numb and once again shut down emotionally. I needed time to process the enormity of this latest development. I simply held her hand and listened while she calmly and concisely repeated the conversation she had had with her GP. Then I wrapped her in my arms while we both struggled to control our raw emotions.

After Shirley left, I sat slumped on my bed in a semi-stupor, watching my hands shake. Gradually the numbness passed and the full implications of this new blow overrode all my defence mechanisms, releasing previously inhibited fears and doubts to drown me in grief. How could I even begin to contemplate my life without this wonderful woman by my side? How would I survive with such an essential part of me – my cherished wife, companion, lover and soulmate – taken from me? And what would it do to our children? They would be faced with the possibility of losing two parents. Too much, Lord, too much.

But, as was often the case, it was Shirley's own example that eventually brought me back to some semblance of calm and acceptance. If she could face each new disappointment and find the courage to continue the fight – to do whatever she believed necessary in order to be obedient to God's will; if she could remain steadfast and maintain her belief that she would be healed when so much evidence negated it; then I must also find the strength to support her and reclaim my own peace.

CHAPTER 13

Why Me, Lord?

Graeme ~ As long as I live, I shall ask the burning question: 'Why me Lord?' Why was I saved and my beloved Shirley taken from us? I am sure many people who watched our saga unfold from the sidelines asked the same unfathomable question. Perhaps it was that God had other plans for Shirley; perhaps He has other plans for me; we may never know the answer. But I do believe God's promise that He will never burden us with a weight too heavy for us to carry.

Monday 9 September 2013

Shirley ~ Today I cancelled my six-weekly appointment with the oncologist. Following the last discouraging appointment, I'm very aware that all he can offer is chemotherapy and I can't bear the thought of taking any more – it is so destructive to my body.

Tuesday 10 September 2013

> How beautiful on the mountains are the feet of those who bring good news, who proclaim peace, who bring good tidings, who proclaim salvation, who say to Zion, 'Your God reigns!' (Isaiah 52:7)

Shirley ~ I've been feeling at a crossroads. I am at such odds that I am struggling with prayer for healing, unsure at this point if that is what I should be asking God for. My quandary is that I am more and more coming to the realisation that praise and worship is the key and I am being drawn to place all my energies in this direction. This choice also keeps me positive and prevents doubts from creeping in when it would be easy to give up.

Knowing how I was feeling, Graeme suggested it was a good time to take another look at our Mission Statement, and after going through it we both felt reinvigorated. While showering, I got to thinking of how beneficial it had been for us to formulate that statement together and I felt inspired to encourage Michelle and Richard to make one as well. As bystanders, this journey has been equally traumatic for them and it could help to clarify their own beliefs about how our family is dealing with the fallout from this insidious disease.

Friday 13 September 2013

Julie ~ I just want you to know I am very much seeking the Lord to show you what is the way for you, so that He can bring forth His miracle in your life however He wants to do that. As you follow His leading, so you will bring honour and praise to Him, for He will bring you through in victory.

Shirley ~ With one very large and some smaller glands up in my neck and supraclavicle area, my mind has been working overtime and I had a darned good cry today. My pain is for Graeme and our children; it is also for those who seem to silently mock our confidence in believing God's Word that He will heal.

With all that in mind, I decided that I should now have the

CT scan that the oncologist has wanted me to have for months. I am tired of second-guessing, and one way or another I really need to have the answers.

I went to bed with a clearer mind – relieved that I had finally made a decision. Then I woke in the middle of the night and lay in a semi-conscious state second-guessing my decision and arguing with myself. And then got to thinking of how my perceptions about this journey have been shaped by circumstances, varied opinions (both medical and biblical), and my own confusion. I've been like a feather swirling in the wind, unable to overcome the elements and determine my own course. I concluded that I really had no choice about the outcome and felt helpless at my total lack of control. Then I remembered a few lines from a self-help book someone gave me that talked about controlling the controllables. It said, in essence, that when there was absolutely nothing you could do about a situation, all you were left with was your own attitude towards it. Light bulb moment: it came to me that the choice I could make was to view this experience as trauma, or as an affliction sent by God to attract my attention to Him. Viewed from this perspective, it all came together and made complete sense.

Sunday 22 September 2013

Shirley – As we read the Bible together this evening we marvelled again at how directly God speaks into our lives:

> 'no weapon forged against you will prevail, and you will refute every tongue that accuses you. This is the heritage of the servants of the LORD, and this is their vindication from me,' declares the LORD. (Isaiah 54:17)

We prayed blessing into the 'c situation' and claimed the protection of the blood of Jesus over each family member.

Julie ~ Declaring complete healing for you both. While praying for you, I pictured those waves of God, washing all cancer and sickness away. He gave that word, He will do it. God sees your faithfulness towards Him, sees when you've been battered. He loves you sooooo much and knows how much of a hard road this has been. He loves your persistence in being faithful to Him. Your house is a house of the Lord. He is first in your lives, your King and your God. Let your praises continue to ring out to Him. You are coming into a new season, a brand new day. Be encouraged.

Monday 23 September 2013

Shirley ~ I woke at 1 a.m. last night with severe, deep, nauseating back pain. Again Graeme and I claimed protection from God and the pain started to abate. An hour and a half later I was clear of pain.

> For God did not give us a spirit of timidity, but a spirit of power, of love and of self-discipline. (2 Timothy 1:7)

Slept soundly, praise the Lord. Why, I wonder, do others not see that these are minor miracles along the way? Does it have to be all or nothing?

In the evening, I attended the prayer meeting at a friend's home. After a few other similar testimonies, I decided to share the above experience with the group. I was thoroughly blessed as some later prayed over our situation.

Seek peace and pursue it. (Psalm 34:14 and 1 Peter 3:11)

Tuesday 24 September 2013

Shirley – Wow how time flies – today marks another year for Michelle. Now she too is a mum, and I am delighting in being able to share some of my child-rearing experiences with her and pass on tips for adapting to their new lifestyle. I think that there is an underlying sense of urgency to get in as much information as possible in the time we have together. And, as is often the case with new mums, Michelle is being inundated with advice from everyone she comes into contact with. Apart from the fact that this is overwhelming, the advice is also very often conflicting, and she laughingly calls me her 'information filter' and trusts my judgement (a lot to do with being her mum, I'm sure, but also supported by my years as a midwife). During our evening ritual of praying for God to bless our children, Graeme passed the baton on to Dale for their children:

> The LORD bless you and keep you; the LORD make his face shine on you and be gracious to you; the LORD turn his face toward you and give you peace. (Numbers 6:24-26)

Today I booked for a CT scan – it's taken four months for me to respond to the request form. Rather an emotional event. After I put the phone down I totally lost the plot and bawled my eyes out. My reluctance is based on not wanting to give potential ammunition to the oncologist regarding more chemotherapy – that seems such a destructive idea with only a 30 to 50 percent chance of effectiveness, and a host of potential side effects. I'm not quite sure about the point of a scan because I don't need any discouragement if a physical manifestation of healing isn't present. It all ties in with the ambiguity Graeme and I feel between medical facts and God's truth.

I told God that I totally trust Him – but 'please help my unbelief'. My faith in God's Word for healing is so strong, yet I know it is as small as a mustard seed. God is my healer. Despite pain in the hip and down to my groin, I press in to closer intimacy with God and knowing His Word.

Following my devotional I read my Bible. I should never doubt for one instance that God is always watching over me and providing me with words of comfort whenever I need them. He gave me such a direct answer to my cry for help:

> O LORD, how many are my foes! How many rise up against me! Many are saying of me, 'God will not deliver him.' But you are a shield around me, O LORD; you bestow glory on me and lift up my head. To the LORD I cry aloud, and he answers me from his holy hill... From the LORD comes deliverance. May your blessing be on your people. (Psalm 3:1-4,8)

Friday 27 September 2013

Julie ~ Shirley, I don't believe that He is taking you home at this time, but just say that was true, what you are doing is right for you – believing in your healing and getting close to God is not wrong. It will always be the right thing to do, no matter what the outcome.

Shirley ~ I guess the beauty of our intimacy with God is that it's not a place to boast or for seeking human attention. It is what it is – time out with God and getting to know HIM more closely.

So maybe it is better if you don't see yourself as needing to be a wonderful example, but maybe God in His infinite wisdom is still using you in that way – His way.

And I know that He is trying to reach me in so many different ways. I am getting better (I think) at looking for clues and listening more closely to His personal messages. Like so many other people (I am sure) I always cherish my reading of *Word for Today*, and I am often blown away by the timing of the message and its significance for me. I particularly love this:

> Now is the time to guard your heart and your mind. Let the Word of God wash your thinking. Read the Bible daily, meditate on it and be transformed by the renewing of your mind. Robert Browning wrote: 'Why stay we on the earth except to grow?' Yet few dedicate themselves to this process. That's because growth requires change, and we are uncomfortable with what change brings. If we don't change we won't grow, and if we don't grow we're not really living. Growth demands a temporary surrender of security. It means giving up familiar but limiting patterns, safe but unrewarding work. Taking a new step is often what we fear most. (*Word for Today*)

Monday 30 September 2013

Shirley ~ CT scan today – I have peace that God is okay with me going ahead with this procedure. The key word today is FAITH.

> And without faith it is impossible to please God, because everyone who comes to him must believe that he exists and that he rewards those who earnestly seek him. By faith Noah, when warned about things not yet seen, in holy fear built an

Peace in the Storm

ark to save his family. By his faith he condemned the world and became heir of the righteousness that comes by faith. (Hebrews 11:6-7)

During the afternoon, my dear husband called the oncology department to try and get the results before I could be told. Then he hurried home to be here when they notified me. That's love, and I appreciate him so much for wanting to protect me from the shock or at least share the impact with me. Medically speaking, it does not look good:

- Cancer is now also in the right breast and axilla – numerous nodes, one measuring 1.3 centimetres. (Last week I noticed that the nipple on my right breast had receded into it.)
- Multiple new metastases in both lobes of the liver. One up to 1.8 centimetres across. Evidence of metastatic disease progression within liver and throughout the imaged skeleton.
- Increase in sclerotic cancerous lesions in spine and bony pelvis.

Words. Words! WORDS! Ominous, cavalier, destructive and – if allowed – annihilating. But God is our shield and we are protected. Satan was defeated once and for all at Calvary. Today Graeme and I declare that God has the VICTORY in our lives. We may be knocked back but we aren't knocked down.

Tuesday 1 October 2013

Shirley ~ I really don't need reminders to love God – that is a given – but sometimes it helps to be reminded that for love to flourish it needs a deepening of intimacy and tangible proof. So it is good to be nudged from time to time with reminders not to take my relationship with God for granted, and to find ways to become even closer to Him.

> Godly character is formed through intimacy with God, and it flows through integrity with people. Intimacy means: 'close familiarity or friendship'. Intimacy with God is God's greatest desire for us … 'Love the Lord your God with all your heart and with all your soul and with all your mind.' (Matthew 22:37) (Steve McCracken)

Wednesday 2 October 2013

Shirley – I initially dismissed the following because 'it wasn't for me'.

> For it has been granted to you on behalf of Christ not only to believe on him, but also to suffer for him… (Philippians 1:29)

> You need the kind of faith that not only believes God for good things, but also sustains you through bad things. The Bible says, 'if you suffer for doing what is right, God will reward you for it. So don't worry or be afraid… Instead… worship Christ as Lord of your life…' (1 Peter 3:14-15 NLT). God has foresight but we have only hindsight. So whether the path you've been called to walk is rough or smooth, your attitude should be one of worship, acknowledging 'Christ as Lord of your life'. Joseph's slavery led to the saving of his

Peace in the Storm

family. The lions' den led Daniel to a cabinet position. Christ entered the world by a surprise pregnancy and redeemed it through an unjust murder. (*Word for Today*)

I'm understanding that God allows suffering, that the verses for example that say 'the angel of the LORD encamps around those who fear him' (Psalm 34:7) and '…under his wings you will find refuge' (Psalm 91:4) don't mean that I am, as a believer, necessarily exempt from the pain in our fallen world. God protects us from Satan's lesser and limited power. God promises to be absolutely so close to me in all circumstances.

The seething emotions over the period following my scan results finally erupted in another crying jag today and left me a rather sad soggy mess. As I hovered over the phone, thinking 'no I shouldn't disturb Graeme at work with a crying wife', it rang. It was a friend calling from Melbourne. As she later said, 'God heard your cry, He knows and understands your situation and how you feel. That's why He prompted me to call. I wish I could be there for you.' To which I replied, 'It doesn't matter where you are, God chose you to be the one to call me right now. He knows what He's doing.' She then followed up the phone call with an email:

> I understand your concern that some Christians would be very discouraged if you were to die of cancer at this point in time, significantly, after so many prayers for your recovery and healing. But God does not need anyone to protect His reputation.
>
> Was God wrong when He said you were healed? No, He was not. But the true meaning of that goes much deeper than our understanding.

Shirley - Abraham, too, sought facts (like me having that CT scan), and when God said that he would be a father of many nations he looked at the 'medical facts' for both him and Sarah and questioned them. But God still blessed him:

> Without weakening in his faith, he faced the fact that his body was as good as dead – since he was about a hundred years old – and that Sarah's womb was also dead. Yet he did not waver through unbelief regarding the promise of God, but was strengthened in his faith and gave glory to God. (Romans 4:19-20)

Julie - No regrets – that you have poured your life out, to the best of your ability, for your faith, your marriage, your husband, children, and for others. This is how we should all live our lives. If you live with this in mind, on a daily basis, there will be no regrets. The first and greatest commandment is being worked out in your life. This was not saying that the end is near. This is saying that God is pleased with the way you have given yourself for the things that are most important, and to continue doing that. For mankind there is no greater love or purpose. Many will envy your commitment to God and family.

Thursday 3 October 2013

> When your thoughts and desires are submitted to Him He will actually think and speak through you. What a privilege. (*Word for Today*)

> Despite all these things, overwhelming victory is ours through Christ... (Romans 8:37 NLT)

Julie ~ Isaiah 46:3-4 spoke to me of God's loving protection over you: 'Listen to me [Shirley]... whom I have upheld since you were conceived, and have carried since your birth. Even to your old age and gray hairs I am He, I am He who will sustain you. I have made you and I will carry you; I will sustain you and I will rescue you.'

Because of who He is you are safe despite all of the evidence. Safe in Jesus' arms ... carried by Him. With all my love, honour and respect, for having shown the world a better way through your own journey.

Shirley ~ I am grateful that God is using what is very traumatic suffering in me, to draw others into a closer, more intimate, walk with Him. What a privilege. God has been showing me that each person is on their own journey and I should not feel responsible for anyone else's perception of the outcome of mine. It is God who allows these things.

Saturday 12 October 2013

Shirley ~ Over the past seven months since finishing the last chemotherapy treatment, I have been blessed with good health – I both look well and feel even better. People regularly remark: 'You are looking so good, how are you feeling?' 'Well, whatever you are doing, Shirley, must be really good.' We serve a wonderful God and Heavenly Father.

> Where does my help come from? My help comes from the Lord, the Maker of heaven and earth. (Psalm 121:1-2)

Our family is under some pressure at the moment, with final

university deadlines in progress for Richard; and my dad, whose health has shown some deterioration this past week, needing hospitalisation. Graeme and I have taken the plunge and booked a trip to Hawaii next week. Mixed feelings about this one. Of course I'd love to have a fabulous holiday away together but we would be abandoning our family when they need us most. Our prayer is that we might see a supernatural intervention and have a visible testimony of God's grace.

There is no change in my stake in the ground. I believe that a physical healing will have little effect on my relationship with God. For most of my Christian life, my relationship with God has NOT been dependent on what He could do for me but rather on WHO HE IS and WHAT HE HAS ALREADY DONE FOR ME AT THE CROSS. At its very core, our relationship is founded on an unshakeable personal awareness and knowledge of the goodness and incomprehensible love of my Heavenly Father; the sure and certain knowledge that Jesus is my Saviour and Lord; and that I have the hope of living in eternity with Him. That won't change regardless of my circumstances.

I long to be here to share the deep truths of our faith. My heart's desire is to walk the grace granted to me, embodying His love and being a living testimony to His power, speaking to the hearts of those who have witnessed my journey.

But interestingly, these longings expose two things: my arrogance in thinking God needs me to accomplish His good purpose; and the challenge to trust my family into His care, knowing He has already designed the course of their lives. My prayer is that the ugliness of my battle with cancer will be used in a meaningful way to shape the hearts of my children, husband and our community.

Saturday 19 – Tuesday 29 October 2013

Shirley – Ten days in Hawaii with my darling husband, thinking it couldn't get much better than this. Not the best start however. Our first night at the Royal Hawaiian on Waikiki Beach, I was in agony with sharp stabbing pains radiating out from my spine and intense stomach pain. At 10 p.m., after five hours, we phoned friends in New Zealand and asked them to pray. As they prayed I immediately started vomiting and continued over the next hour. By midnight, the back pain was unrelieved, so Graeme sought help and we were taxied to a local medical centre. As we drove, the pain began to subside, and by the time we reached hospital, it had virtually gone. I felt rather a fraud.

Nevertheless, the doctor and nurse were extremely supportive and friendly. After following through admission procedures, they concluded there was something wrong with my gall bladder. Uh-oh, an ultrasound showed nothing wrong. Another few dollars tallied up. I was flouting all the doom and gloom predictions of the medical fraternity. The staff said that by now my legs should have atrophied and I'd be in a wheelchair, and incontinent. Moreover, staying well for the next ten days in Hawaii seemed an impossible feat to them: 'So come back again when you need us.' Returned to our room by 3 a.m.

Well, the truth is I did stay well. Next day after a sleep in, Graeme and I hired a car and drove around the west side of Oahu, past the world famous surfing destination; visited the Dole pineapple plantation; then Waimea Valley Botanical Garden, where we opted out of a trek down to the waterfall, 'slightly' weary after the previous evening's experience.

On the way back, I was talking to God about my current situation. Yesterday I thought that my good days were finished.

Yet here I was, mobile again and pain free. Weird? It can only be a miracle. 'Lord, what is going on?' 'I will heal you.' 'When?' 'Wait.' 'God show me only your truth please. Save me from wild imaginings.'

Just two more episodes of similar back pain over the next few evenings, but all the days were pain free. Fit and well enough to thoroughly enjoy exploring both Oahu and Maui islands (in our rental Mustang V6 – not quite up to the standard of Graeme's V8 muscle car). Thank you, Lord.

On the last night, which happened to be our twenty-fourth wedding anniversary, our thoughtful travel agent had organised a catamaran cruise. During the evening, all honeymooners and those with anniversaries were invited to the dance floor. As we danced I had a premonition: 'this could be our last wedding anniversary,' and fought to control my tears.

Graeme ~ Memories are made of this. The simple pleasure of dancing cheek to cheek with someone you love; holding her familiar body close, with our contours fitting together in relaxed intimacy as we moved to the music. And as the rhythm moved up-tempo, swinging her out and drowning in her sparkling brown eyes. It was as if we were in a world of our own, and it wasn't until someone mentioned it might be 'the last dance' that I was reminded of the transience of such moments.

Shirley ~ During our Hawaiian holiday I thought more about the Mary/Martha theme. Where is God when I am suffering? Clearly He had a different prescience to mine. For if I had been healed in 2010 when first diagnosed, I would have been ecstatic and carried on with my full and satisfying life, missing out on myriads of learning curves. Prime example: after the initial breast surgery, chemotherapy and radiotherapy I was determined to step back into my original shoes and move on as usual, which I did. Yes, I had made many changes and adjustments: I learnt a lot from God and His Word; shared words and revelations with others; researched the subject of cancer and possible causes; and used my own experiences to help others going through similar procedures. If I had been healed at that stage, I would have moved on having learnt a lot but still not really recognising the 'Mary' situation in my life.

Then – shock, horror – 18 months after the initial diagnosis, I was faced with the fact that the aggressive cancer was now in multiple spots in my chest wall, lumbar-thoracic spine and bony pelvis. This was devastating news, to say the least. If God had healed me then, I would have been overwhelmingly grateful to Him, but once again life would have continued as usual – although leaving me more aware of God's presence and power in my life.

So here I am now in October 2013 being diagnosed with the further spread of cancer to my liver and right breast. And at the same time I am still filling my days with 'Martha'. Would you believe it? Will I never learn? Where is my 'Mary' time? Seriously!

Landing back at Auckland International Airport was the perfect metaphor for our current situation. We had escaped the reality of our life, living on a natural high for a few magical days, and had now landed back with a jolt into the thick of it. Time to face the realities of the heart-rending decisions needing to be made regarding further treatments.

CHAPTER 14

Tried as by Fire

Thursday 7 November 2013

> In this you greatly rejoice, though now for a little while you may have had to suffer grief in all kinds of trials. These have come so that your faith – of greater worth than gold, which perishes even though refined by fire – may be proved genuine and may result in praise, glory and honour when Jesus Christ is revealed. (1 Peter 1:6-7)

Shirley ~ We attended a radiotherapy planning appointment this evening with regard to treatment for the right breast tumour. As the tumour isn't painful, the oncologist focused on my yellow skin and eyes, saying that my liver looks like it is obstructed and would probably take me out before the breast tumour had a chance. Couldn't be any blunter than that. So an urgent CT scan and blood tests were organised for the following day.

Saturday 9 November 2013

Shirley ~ The 'prophet of doom and gloom' oncologist (poor man, he is a very good person who takes no pleasure from this) has said enough words of death to cause a dark shadow over me.

It is so very hard to open my eyes fully and I feel a bit like giving up. Graeme and I prayed the blood of Jesus over the death sentence pronounced on Thursday, and immediately the shadow lifted and my eyes opened normally. God is amazing. He fills us with such peace.

Graeme ~ Shirley had a keen sense of humour and the ability to laugh at herself. These characteristics played an important role in keeping us all sane while everything around us felt like insanity. As a family, we developed a macabre approach to things that were too close emotionally to be dealt with head-on. I recall the time we all sat around the dinner table in fits of laughter, discussing burial options. It was unanimously agreed that Shirley could not possibly have anything ordinary, and we suggested that our grandfather clock might be a good fit. I opted to be buried in my Ford Mustang. We continued to talk about the 'chemo diet' as a weight-loss method, and when Shirley began to show obvious signs of jaundice, she called it her 'Hawaiian tan'.

Monday 11 November 2013

Shirley ~ Another appointment with the 'prophet of doom and gloom'. This time we were being well covered against subsequent feelings of depression by our prayer group and other wonderful friends. The CT scan results showed very little further spread of the cancer – in fact the bone and chest wall appeared stabilised. Lungs clear, praise the Lord. The bile ducts' walls showed thickening and a build up of bile was dilating the ducts in behind the obstruction. Causes could be inflammation ('but you are looking far too well for that to be the cause') or cancer, which is strangely presumed to be the culprit.

Fairly urgent course of action with two options: (a) stents inserted into the two offending ducts, the procedure done under sedation and internally through the mouth to stomach to gall bladder; or (b) a drainage tube permanently inserted to remove the bile and bypass the blockage. Over the next day, the gastro-enterologist will be in contact.

After the appointment, the prayer group leader reported that their meeting (which had been held at the same time) was full of praising and thanking God for who He is and what He is doing in my life. There was a wonderful sense of God's anointing on the group.

Tuesday 12 November 2013

Julie ~ Reading *Waking the Dead* by John Eldredge. The theme of the book is that we need to wake up and come to our senses, and realise that we are actors in a critical drama and have a vital role to play. It is just so very true and relates, I think, specifically to you. I quote:

> You are not what you think you are. There is a glory to your life that your enemy fears, and he is hell-bent on destroying that glory before you act on it. But once you begin to see with the eyes of your heart, once you have begun to know it is true from the bottom of your heart, it will change every-thing. The story of your life is the story of the long and brutal assault on your heart by the one who knows what you could be and fears it.

Love you, Girl. You are my champion. I thank God every time I think of you during the day. For your strong faith and the courage you show to fight the 'little c' with the strength of your 'BIG C' – Christ in you, the hope of glory.

Shirley – Dear friends, as a family we appreciate your prayers, love and care. We are emphatic when we say again that 'All the days ordained for me were written in your book before one of them came to be.' (Psalm 139:16) We rest in that.

> Just as a diamond is formed from common carbon placed under pressure of over a million tons per square metre – so the character of Christ is formed in you by adverse circumstances. When Paul thought he couldn't stand anymore, God told him: 'My grace is sufficient for you…' (2 Corinthians 12:9) (*Word for Today*)

Thursday 14 November 2013

Graeme – Shirley and I had discussed the inevitability of her missing out on milestones in Richard's life, such as marriage and children, and she was deeply saddened by that thought. She wanted to do something for Richard, here and now, to mark some achievement in his life; something that he could remember as being a special time spent with his mum and family all together. So we came up with the idea of having an End of University celebration.

Tuesday 19 November 2013

Shirley – Today at Auckland Hospital for an ERCP (endoscopic retrograde cholangiopancreatography) to insert a stent through the malignant growth that blocks my common bile duct. As noted by the surgeon, post-operatively, 'It was a complex and difficult procedure owing to patient discomfort.' Well, thanks to his sedation, which was supposed to be limited because of some liver dysfunction, I don't remember anything. Quite a lot of discomfort afterwards though, where the procedure was carried out, and some analgesia required but mostly my body is very weary from struggling with the raised blood bile levels (bilirubin) at 250 (normal being 0 to 20).

Wednesday 20 November 2013

Shirley ~ It's always a relief to be on the other side of these procedures – I am so over them. Light glimmers through all this darkness from time to time, and it comes as a result of the constant prayers said on our behalf. Small but significant things become a blessing, like having an unusually good, natural night's sleep; avoiding the extreme after-effects and reactions normally experienced by people undergoing similar procedures; and the no small miracle that the narrow gauge wire was able to guide a plastic stent through the six centimetre stricture in my main common bile duct, saving the alternative of a permanent drainage tube from inside the abdomen to the exterior.

The increasing toxic build-up of bile in my bloodstream has left me pretty wasted and sleepy. It is great news that the stent was functioning well; however, here comes the BUT: we are reminded that a plastic stent is only temporary and will probably block in six weeks to three months, requiring a repeat procedure. With a malignant cause of obstruction, we were given a pretty clear impression that this length of time was probably all that was required. Well, we intend to consult with the Great Physician on that one.

The initial back pain experienced post-procedure appeared to be from my bony spine, but as time went on it was clear to the surgeon that it was from the stent and gall bladder area, and I could feel it radiating into my back. Today, thankfully, pain has been minimal, requiring no analgesia.

So life keeps going and we give God all the glory no matter what. He is sovereign and we trust Him. We are blessed with amazingly supportive family and friends.

Friday 29 November 2013

Shirley ~ My emotions continue to be buffeted by conflicting advice and the vagaries of my own tortured soul. I swing from a point of being resigned to fulfilling God's plan for me and accepting whatever pathway He wants to lead me on, to being filled with a knowing that I will be healed and having this viewpoint reinforced by others. For example, this evening at our weekly prayer meeting, I was presented with these words: 'Be still and know that I am the Lord who heals you.' Is it any wonder I am confused?

Julie ~ 'Certainly God has heard me; he has attended to the voice of my prayer.' (Psalm 66:19 NKJV) Your faith is amazing. I have been reading through 1 Peter where it talks about this present suffering in the world – it is temporary and considered necessary by God to prove our faith genuine, resulting in praise, glory and honour when Jesus comes again. Keep going – God will show you the way, even when there seems to be no way. You are amazing.

Graeme ~ In the midst of all this, I felt extremely uncomfortable about thinking of myself, but genuinely concerned friends had been enquiring about the result of a CT scan I had just undergone. So I sent off a quick note:

> Just letting you know the surgeon is very happy with my progress and says there are no signs of cancer anywhere and my joins are all well sealed. So praise the Lord. I still have some odd bowel motions (very frequent followed by very infrequent), but apparently that will gradually improve over the next year and then settle into a new normal. Who knows what that will be? I have one more out of 10 sponsored Steel Pilates sessions left – designed to assist men who have had cancer to get back physical strength, balance and muscle tone. It is the equivalent of Pink Pilates for women, which was of great benefit to Shirley.

I'll never know what others really thought about the contradictions of our situation. Perhaps by focusing on my healing they were not required to delve too deeply into the other half of our equation. Logically, they were experiencing the same swinging emotions and conflicting beliefs as we did – none of us know how we will react when placed in such intolerable circumstances and we can only do what we perceive to be the 'right' thing at the time. By this stage in the journey we were wondering, what exactly constitutes healing? To Shirley, healing was never based on the 'all or nothing' concept but viewed as a catalyst to bring her to a closer relationship with God.

Friday 6 December 2013

Shirley – Ever had itchy feet? That seems to be one small area of expertise I failed to pick up during my nursing career. Over the last week, I've become suspicious that the bile duct stent, inserted during surgery two and a half weeks ago, isn't draining adequately. Those itchy feet again, plus a number of other symptoms: continued jaundice and extreme lethargy. Today blood results came through indicating that my bilirubin levels are becoming high and toxic again. So an appointment with the gastroenterologist on Saturday will no doubt lead to further investigations and decisions. Can't wait!

Yesterday I started 12 daily doses (excluding weekends) of radiotherapy to the axilla, right breast and collar bone area. In 2010 I was given 25 daily doses; this time the same amount of radiation will be in the 12 doses. We have decided that it is reasonable to go through with this to try and kick back the tumour growth.

Yes, we truly appreciate the many alternative ideas that have been suggested, like taking flaxseed oil and cottage cheese, only eating unprocessed food, or consuming large amounts of asparagus, and numerous other innovative cures. In all probability these ideas have merit and just maybe they do hold the answer to curing cancer. Perhaps someday someone else will prove they are right and get them researched. Of course we don't think that further radiotherapy is ideal, but we're running out of options.

All of the above wasn't too positive I know. But still we press into the power of our mighty God, knowing everything is in His hands and we trust Him. Despite natural human emotions, our family is being sustained by His constant peace and inner strength. And I am even more grateful when I think of the incredible pain and misery of others we have met, dear folk who have little or no family support, who give up without the hope of eternity with a loving God. We realise how blessed we are to be in His family, to have strength and focus outside of ourselves.

Monday 9 December 2013

Shirley – Well, it seems to have reached the eleventh hour. Sometimes this situation is so unreal – so incomprehensible it seems a delusion, like a badly scripted movie or a very bad nightmare I will wake up from. But I know it is real – all of it – and it is too late to rewrite the ending.

In the ultrasound scan on Monday it was discovered that the bile duct stent was still in place, there was minimal accumulation of fluid behind the stents but many blockages by tumours within the liver. This time the right pleural cavity (around my lung) was seen to have 400 ml+ fluid, explaining the persistent cough and breathlessness. But it seemed like I had no medic to coordinate the decisions now required. The recent gastroenterologist I had seen for the stent wasn't into the thoracic cavity for pleural drainage; the radiotherapist was too specialised; the chemotherapy oncologist is on a 12-day holiday, and I guess he has been the main coordinator. It felt like I was falling between the cracks and no one cared. At which point I was told by ultrasound radiologist to phone the hospice.

Resigned, I did as instructed. And found, despite my preconceived ideas earlier in the year about their purpose being just to look after the terminally ill, that they were far more than that; a very caring compassionate group of people, full of helpful resources; so very different to the clinical hospital situation. So an appointment was set up for Graeme and me with the hospice physician, our case nurse and the family support person. Whoa. Clearly they had done their research before the meeting. I so appreciate their competence. But what they said was enough to shake us to the very core.

The bile duct stent (inserted three weeks ago) is blocked. To perform an alternate drainage to the outside would probably only be temporary and the chances of infection following surgery are very high considering my weakened body state. I would be in Auckland Hospital for a week.

Last year I had a successful left pleurodesis ('gluing' procedure of lung to chest wall to eliminate the pleural cavity). The newly found 400 millilitres of pleural effusion on the right side explains my persistent cough over the last few weeks. It also explains the awful breathlessness I'm having at times. We fully expected that the medical staff would organise fluid drainage, but apparently with existing liver damage the chance of haemorrhage is too high for the procedure. Radiotherapy – discontinue this – it's only a temporary band-aid that carries unpleasant side-effects I don't need.

Conclusion: It was years, then months, then weeks. Yesterday an indication of the severity of the situation is that they are now talking days (perhaps a few weeks). The toxicity of the bile in my blood to my body organs is high and I'm struggling. But I seriously don't feel like I'm dying. Maybe because I've never experienced it before and have no idea how I 'should' be feeling. Is there a check-list?

Friday 13 December 2013

Graeme ~ Shirley never conceded that cancer had ravaged her life. She coped with whatever was thrown at her and just kept going. She was a survivor. She always managed to find something encouraging in every disappointment – she worked on a relativity basis, saying it could have been worse; if one treatment didn't work there would be another that might. And she kept believing that at some point she would win this battle. But even for her there were times when tenacity didn't cut it and it was faith and faith alone that kept her going. And at her lowest ebb she still put concern for others before her own. At this point, she sent out what was to be her last email, bringing everyone up to date and demonstrating to the end that she was still in a positive frame of mind:

Shirley ~ Oh how we all appreciate your love and support. We have also had my brother and sister-in-law staying from Dunedin for a couple of nights, and it was so, so good, to have them right there to see and touch. Close family bonding is such a blessing and makes you feel so very cared for and loved – I, of course, savoured every moment.

We have also had a heap of stuff going on with my dad. Michelle has shown amazing dedication transporting a rather unsteady Grandad to appointments, but I know how much he loves being in her company and appreciates everything she does for him. He has decided to move to the rest home section of the retirement village where he lives, so we planned a meeting with the manager. This is a constructive step for him and a relief for the family knowing he will be well cared for.

I am pretty exhausted. But we all acknowledge that God is so much in this and every situation. God's peace reigns in our home. He wants a relationship with each of us more than anything else on the planet.

Julie ~ I appreciate your honesty, humour and brightness in a situation that leaves us with many questions. Your comments about family, support and hope are a real testimony in themselves.

Where would we be without a loving Father orchestrating our lives for our good? All the best dear Shirley, as day by day you walk by faith. I believe your testimony will bless many and bring glory to God.

Epilogue

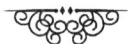

Shirley's account of her journey began with her first email on Thursday 20 May 2010 and ended with her final instalment written on Friday 13 December 2013.

Her physical strength lessened as time progressed and she spent much of it sitting in a lounge chair surrounded by people who loved her. She enjoyed Christmas dinner with our wider family and came with us to Pauanui in early January. Shirley's determination that we should have this happy memory of a last family holiday together reflected her unselfish love for us.

Another way she expressed her love was through the legacy letters she wrote for Michelle, Richard and Dale.

Precious Michelle, I love you so so much. Over 23 years ago I held my beautiful baby girl for the first time and was overcome with pride and joy. There was never any doubt about what we would call you; the meaning of your name is 'A gift from God'. I am so proud of you – in every area of your life you have set a high bar and always cleared it. I am confident that you chose the best possible husband in Dale and that God has always directed your choices. You have been a wonderful daughter, and when I see you with Jasmine I know that you will bring her up to have the same values and integrity, love and compassion, and reap the same rewards as I have with you. I leave the three of you in God's loving hands. xxx

Hey Rich. Twenty-two years ago a bundle of utter joy came into the world and completed our wonderful family unit. And you have kept us entertained and enthralled from the moment you were born. You enriched our lives with great conversation, entertaining stories, and were always just plain good fun company – who wouldn't like you? I wouldn't change a moment of it – it's been a brilliant 22 years and I give thanks to God for bringing you into my life. I love you because you're the absolute best son God could have ever given me. xxx

Dale, thanks for being a fantastic son-in-law and I know that you will also be a wonderful father to your precious new baby girl. You and Michelle have a strong foundation in your lives – Christian families and early personal commitments of your own lives to God, as well as wonderful friends. You have been granted the gift of interdependence with each other and God. You, like Michelle, have been given the wings to fly through life with great moral values and personal choices. These things have made you the people you are today. The Bible says that 'A cord of three strands is not quickly broken.' As God is the centre of your marriage and family, of all your decisions, so He will honour and bless you.

In accordance with Shirley's wishes, and in total agreement with our own (supported by Hospice and the district nurse), we were able to care for her at home. We prayed she would have a sound mind, and apart from some minor lapses, which she

Epilogue

would usually pick up herself and laugh about, Shirley remained lucid and aware of events until the end. Hospice had offered, if she wished, to ensure she would be in 'dreamland' and not endure any pain or sense of 'this is it'. But she was very emphatic that we walk this journey together – with our Lord God – and not be in a chemical daze.

On the evening of Sunday 19 January 2014, we held a family prayer time: 'God, if it is not your will for Shirley/Mum to be healed this side of heaven, then please have mercy on her and allow her to pass from this world soon. Please don't allow her to continue like this.' Up until this time Shirley had spent her days in a La-Z-Boy in the lounge, able to speak and hold conversations, however from Monday morning she remained in bed. There was a significant decline in movement and she could respond only by squeezing our hands.

On Wednesday, Shirley's breathing was heavy but steady. Although no longer speaking, she still understood and would acknowledge us or what we said to her with a slight raise of her eyebrows. Separately, we each (Shirley's father, Richard, Michelle and myself) were able to tell her that we were letting go of her from this world and that she could die with the peace of that knowledge. 'I love you and I want you to be here, more than anything – but not like this. We will look after each other; I'm okay for you to go now,' I told her.

On the evening of Wednesday 22 January 2014, aged 61, Shirley passed from our world, safe in the arms of her Saviour and God.

For us, the physical separation by death is for a season, as we think of Shirley having 'crossed a river' to heaven, where she is totally healed and living in paradise. We are just on either side of the river.

Peace in the Storm

Right until her last breath, Shirley had a genuine and complete peace, which came from the knowledge that she could say with certainty:

> I have fought the good fight, I have finished the race, I have kept the faith. Now there is in store for me the crown of righteousness, which the Lord, the righteous Judge, will award to me on that day… (2 Timothy 4:7-8)

God used her journey through cancer to produce in her the nature of Jesus, as God's plan is to change people and not necessarily situations.

Dear Reader

If your heart has been opened while reading Shirley's story, and you have been touched by her amazing faith, and would like to explore how a personal relationship with God can bring purpose, power, peace and pardon into your life, I would love to hear from you. Graeme Danco: dyinggraciously@gmail.com

Glossary of Terms

acid reflux – acid from the stomach rises into the lower end of the gullet (oesophagus) and causes burning pain.

adenocarcinoma – a type of cancerous tumour in tissue that has glandular origin, glandular characteristics, or both.

anal fissure – linear tear of the lining of the anal canal.

analgesia – pain relief medication.

anti-emetics / anti-nauseous medication – medicines to reduce nausea and vomiting.

axilla – armpit.

axillary lymph nodes – lymph nodes in the armpit collect infectious or tumour material from nearby to help the body mount an immune response. Breast cancer most commonly spreads to lymph nodes in the arm pit.

bile duct – the tubular structure that drains bile from the liver into the intestine.

bilirubin – a yellow breakdown product found in the liver and blood. When levels are high, people become jaundiced and elevated levels may indicate certain diseases.

bowel cancer – malignant tumour of the intestine, usually the large intestine.

carotid artery – artery bringing blood from the heart to the brain.

catheter – a tube used for the transfer of fluids. Most commonly a urinary cable to drain urine from the bladder into a bag.

Capecitabine – a chemotherapy drug.

chemotherapy – a cancer treatment that uses chemical substances, especially one or more anti-cancer drugs, that target cancer cells.

colorectal tumour – a growth found in the large intestine. Such growths may be benign or malignant (cancerous).

CT scan – computed tomography, an imagining procedure that produce cross-sectional images of the body using x-rays and a computer.

Cyclophosphamide – a chemotherapy drug.

dermal lymph layer – small drainage vessels in the skin.

Dexamethazone (intravenous) – a steroid (to reduce swelling and inflammation) given via the veins (rather than by mouth).

DVT (deep vein thrombosis) – clots in the deep veins, usually in the legs.

Epirubicin – a chemotherapy drug.

ERCP – endoscopic retrograde cholangiopancreatography.

Fluorouracil – a chemotherapy drug.

GP – general practitioner.

Gray – a unit of measure for doses of radiation delivered to the body, usually as part of cancer treatment.

Herceptin – a targeted drug therapy for a particular type of breast cancer.

histology results – report made by a pathologist after examining a biopsy specimen.

ileostomy bag – plastic bag specially designed to fit on the site where the intestine is joined to the abdominal wall, which collects intestinal waste.

imaged skeleton – pictures of the human skeleton taken in the x-ray department.

infused – caused to flow into the body, often intravenously.

intubation – placing a tube, often in the upper airway, to allow ventilation

IV antibiotics – intravenous medication to fight infection.

IV infusion – intravenous solution delivered into a person's veins.

jaundice – yellowness caused by the accumulation of bilirubin in a person's body.

jugular vein – large vein in the neck.

lobes of the liver – the liver is made up of left, right, caudate and quadrate lobes.

lumbar thoracic vertebrae – the vertebrae are a series of bones jointly called the spine. The uppermost vertebrae are called cervical, the middle vertebrae are the thoracic and the lower ones are lumbar.

lymphoedema massage – a massage that attempts to reduce limb swelling caused by the accumulation of fluid that occurs because lymphatics are blocked.

lymphoma – cancer of the lymph nodes and cells.

malignant – a very virulent or infectious growth or disease that can spread and eventually cause death.

mammogram – an x-ray of the breast which can reveal cancers.

metastases / metastatic – cancer that has spread beyond the primary site.

morphine – a strong pain relieving medicine of the narcotic class of drugs.

MRI – magnetic resonance imaging. An alternative to other 3D imaging techniques such as CT scanning or ultrasound.

nodes – in particular, lymph nodes, which are common sites to which cancer can spread.

palliative treatment – treatment aimed at relieving symptoms and not curing the disease.

pelvic ileum – the pelvis is made of three bones; the ischium, the ileum and the pubis. The ileum is the wing-like bone at the back of the pelvis.

peripheral neuropathy – damage to the nerves supplying the areas of the body outside the brain and spine. Often caused by toxic drugs such as chemotherapy. Results in pain, numbness and/or weakness.

pleura – the thin layer of cells that cover the outside surface of the lungs and the inside surface of the chest wall. Fluid that collects in between those layers is called pleural fluid or a pleural effusion.

pleural cavity drainage – removing fluid that has accumulated in the pleural cavity (around the lungs).

pleurodesis – placement of an irritating substance in the pleural cavity to cause obliteration of the pleural space to prevent pleural fluid from re-accumulating.

pneumonia – infection in the lung.

port-a-cath – a device placed (surgically) under the skin of the chest wall and connected to a large vein that allows ready access to withdraw blood or infuse drugs or fluids.

Prednisone – a steroid drug.

prognosis – medical outlook.

prophylactic – preventative treatment.

radiation/radiotherapy – use of high energy x-rays to kill dividing cells, such as those in a cancer.

redivac drainage – suction drainage.

right clavicle – right collarbone.

sclerotic cancerous lesions – cancer that has spread to bones and caused increased bone density.

sclerotic spots – x-ray images of sclerotic cancerous lesions.

seroma – a collection of serum, usually beneath a surgical wound.

Glossary

spontaneous pneumothorax – collapse of the lung occurring without external injury.

stent – a rigid supporting tube, usually placed to keep an existing tubular structure open (e.g. an arterial stent or an biliary stent).

steroids – a class of drugs, the commonest in use being corticosteroids, used to reduce inflammation.

stricture – a narrowing.

suppositories – medicines introduced via the rectum.

supraclavicular gland – a lymph node just above the collarbone.

tachycardia – a fast heart beat.

Taxotere – a chemotherapy drug.

tracheotomy – a cut into the windpipe, often used to place a tube to assist with breathing.

tumour marker blood test – a blood test that measure proteins made by cancer cells. Such tests help detect cancers or measure cancer response to treatment.

Vinorelbine – a chemotherapy drug.

Bible copyright and quote permissions

Quotes from the *Believing in You Daily Devotional* by Steve McCracken of David McCracken Ministries, and quotes from *The Word For Today* published by Rhema Media Incorporated are used by permission of the respective publishers. Note: Some quotes are slightly reworded, as recorded by Shirley in her diaries.

Free copies of *The Word For Today* devotional can be obtained from Rhema Media.

All scripture quotations, unless otherwise indicated, are taken from the Holy Bible, New International Version®, NIV®. Copyright © 1973, 1978, 1984, 2011 by Biblica, Inc.™ Used by permission of Zondervan. All rights reserved worldwide. www.zondervan.com. The "NIV" and "New International Version" are trademarks registered in the United States Patent and Trademark Office by Biblica, Inc.™

Scripture quotations marked (NKJV) taken from the New King James Version®. Copyright © 1982 by Thomas Nelson, Inc. Used by permission. All rights reserved.

Scripture quotations marked (KJV) are taken from The Authorized (King James) Version. Rights in the Authorized Version in the United Kingdom are vested in the Crown. Reproduced by permission of the Crown's patentee, Cambridge University Press.

Scripture quotations marked (NRSV) are taken from New Revised Standard Version Bible, copyright © 1989 National Council of the Churches of Christ in the United States of America. Used by permission. All rights reserved.

Scripture quotations marked (NLT) are taken from the Holy Bible, New Living Translation, copyright ©1996, 2004, 2007, 2013 by Tyndale House Foundation. Used by permission of Tyndale House Publishers, Inc., Carol Stream, Illinois 60188. All rights reserved.

www.ingramcontent.com/pod-product-compliance
Lightning Source LLC
Chambersburg PA
CBHW071349290426
44108CB00014B/1482